I0450516

The CDO Diet & Weight Loss Plan!

The Right Plan for Personal Weight Loss!

All Rights Reserved – 2015 CDO

Disclaimer

The material in this publication is designed and intended for informational purposes. It is not intended to be a medical reference or treatment guide. We suggest throughout the book that everyone make their doctor part of their weight loss efforts. We strongly encourage you to show your medical professional this book and a copy of your weight loss plan prior to commencing such program. Everyone is different and everyone will get different results. We are not doctors nor do we consider ourselves medical authorities. Not everything in this book will pertain to everyone and it is up to the individual and their medical representative to determine which parts may apply to their particular situation. The writers and publishers of this book take no responsibility for the application or use of any or all parts of this book. In other words, use common sense, do your research and consult your doctor before and throughout your weight loss.

Contents

Introduction

At some point in our lives, almost everyone has felt the need or desire to lose weight. It might be just a few pounds or maybe even several hundred pounds. The reason might have been to feel better, look better or maybe to help with a medical condition that your weight is contributing to.

Whatever the reason might be, the fact remains that you will need some kind of plan or course of action to make it happen. These things do not happen by themselves and they do not happen overnight. There is no magic bullet or magic wand to wave and the weight flies off never to be seen again.

We are sorry to burst your bubble but the fact remains that in order to lose the weight you have accumulated over the years, something must change. The good news is that this change does not have to be traumatic or heart wrenching.

It need not involve crushing sacrifice or sweat pouring off your head from vigorous exercise.

The reality is that we can achieve a lot with some very easy and minor adjustments to our lifestyle. We can do this all with huge sacrifice and massive amounts of exercise. In fact, we don't WANT to have these two things in any parts of our lives for one simple reason.

They just don't work!

Most of us try like hell to avoid anything truly unpleasant. I'm not talking about spending the afternoon with annoying Aunt Mildred or something like that but rather the things we do each and every day that we do not like or enjoy. We might start down that route but pretty soon we will be looking for detours!

Throughout this book we will be discussing what we need to do to make this work and make it work well. I think you will be pleasantly surprised to see how easy all this can be.

I will say for the first time something that will be repeated throughout this book:

DO EVERYTHING THE SAFE
AND HEALTHY WAY!

I'm not a doctor and I haven't played one on TV, either. Instead, I am a person just like you and everyone else who just found and developed a plan that works. It worked for me and it will work for you if you give it a chance.

But please, check with your doctor before starting any weight loss/exercise program. Everyone is different and not everyone can do everything safely.

So make your doctor your partner. Involve your doctor in every part of your plan and schedule follow-up appointments throughout your weight loss.

It just makes sense to do that. Plus, when you see your overall health improve, that is one heck of a motivating factor!

Everything in this publication is focused on two basic goals. To provide you with the best possible chance of success and to accomplish everything in a healthy and responsible way.

A Little Background

Before we get started, I think it is smart to tell you a little bit about myself. I feel that this is important because a lot of people believe that they cannot successfully lose weight. It is just too difficult, they do not have enough, or any, will power or that they are just too old or too far out of shape.

Well, think again…………………

As I write this I am almost 60 years old. I have always been overweight and have always struggled with my weight. Over the decades a few pounds her and a few pounds there have added up to a LOT of extra weight over the years.

I have and have had my share of health related issues such as high blood pressure, high cholesterol and other issues. The worst of those "other issues" is that I am a Type 2 Diabetic.

For those of you who do not know what a type 2 Diabetic is, that is someone whose body makes some insulin but not enough to properly control the amount of sugar in the bloodstream. This is not something I was born with but acquired roughly 10 years ago.

Though it is not 100% certain exactly who gets Type 2 and who doesn't, it is largely attributed to diet and weight. Not all heavy or overweight people are diabetic but a lot of overweight people are. It's just one of the universal accepted causes.

Over the years my blood sugar would rise and they would adjust my medicines or add another pill. As we get older, things in our bodies work less efficiently than they did when we were younger and this is one of the results. So I began taking more and more medications.

According to my doctor, weight and exercise play an important role in managing blood sugar levels. Anyone who knows me would definitely say that exercise and my name were rarely mentioned in the same sentence. But at this point, it would also be fair to say that managing blood sugar was a big part of my motivation.

Now I should also tell you that I was never a big workout person. I joined a gym one year and tried and had some success but then I had to stop to have some surgery done and I never went back. It took too long driving there and back and working all of that into my schedule. Plus, to be honest, the time thing was just a reason to stop doing what I really didn't enjoy.

I also experience what some might call "senior moments" although not of the mental variety. These "moments" were times I tried to do something I used to do with ease and found out I couldn't do it anymore. That can be a sobering experience and for some, a little hard to accept.

I do not try to act younger (at least not physically) but I also refuse to use that as an excuse anymore. I do not want to sit in front of the TV or computer all day long regardless of the reason.

Another part of my motivation also comes from the fact that I am getting older and I do not want to get to the point where daily activities wear me out or stop me from doing the things that I love. I also do not wish to hasten my need to depend upon others. I figure that the more I manage to do now to lose some weight and improve my physical well being, the longer I will be able to do more things for myself.

If you were to sum up my motivation for doing the things that I do, I would say that it was 50% health reasons and wanting to live longer and 50% just wanting to feel better and do the things I like as long as possible.

I made myself a goal in my later 50's to be in better physical shape when I turned 60 than I was when I hit 50. I kind of think that I am close to hitting that goal but to be honest, the bar wasn't set all that high.

I had neglected my health and physical condition for decades because I was able to. I was blessed with good health so I was always able to do the things I wanted.

But as you get older those things change.

So by now I hope you realize that I am more like you than you might have originally thought. I'm not one of those guys with a 24 inch waist on TV telling you how to look great and live longer. I'm just someone how found a very easy yet effective way to accomplish the same things but in much easier ways.

So, I am not special. I am like everyone else out there and maybe even a bit behind the curve when it comes to physical conditioning. But that's OK because if I could do it, there is absolutely no way you can't!

Your Motivation

Before we get started, we need to figure something out. We need to understand exactly why you want to lose weight. This is important because if we don't know why we are doing something we are far more likely to give up.

The main thing I want to impress upon you if that it has to be YOU that wants to lose weight. If you are doing it because someone else wants you to, you likely will not have much long term success. Even if there are outside factors like health issues driving this change if YOU don't truly wish to lose weight this is not going to work very well.

Our brains need to understand WHY we are doing something and WHAT we are getting out of the effort. It has to be something WE value and that WE want. Not because our spouse or friends want it, but because WE want it. Even a serious medical issue might not be enough if YOU do not really want to lose the weight.

It Has To Be YOU That Wants This!
NOT Someone Else!!!

I am not saying that a spouses request might not be enough or that you will fail if you are doing this for someone else. What I am saying is that unless WE want to do something, we will often look for the first chance to give up or stop what we are doing. Weight loss is no different than most other things in life. There will be times when things go great and the weight comes off and other times when we might get frustrated because nothing seems to do any good. It is during those hard times that we need to be motivated to keep on going!

Look back on some of the past event in your life when you were forced to do something you didn't want to do. How successful were you in those situations? Did you do your best? Probably not. Did you try your hardest? Probably not. When things got tough, did you bail out? Yeah, you probably did.

This doesn't mean you are weak or that you can't do something. It just means that you really didn't have a great desire to do it in the first place. In order to be successful we have to WANT to be successful. We need to understand WHY we want to do something.

At this point it should be said that NEED is not the same as WANT. We might NEED to lose weight or stop smoking, but if we really don't want to, it's not going to happen.

I can speak from experience because when I was first diagnosed with diabetes, I was told that weight was an important factor and that both weight loss and exercise would help me keep the disease under control.

So that in itself was a legitimate and powerful need. But the fact was that I hated exercise and loved a good hamburger and a plate of fries to go with it so nothing really happened. There was a need but no real desire. You need the desire to go along with it.

Another situation that doesn't really work is losing weight because someone else wants you to. It might work if you wanted to make that person happy and that became your motivation but doing something because someone else wants you to. It has to be YOU that wants it not someone else.

It sometimes helps to understand why you want to do something and the benefits you think you will get when you achieve your intended goal.

For example, if you want to lose weight so you will look better for your wedding, then picture yourself in your wedding gown or tuxedo all thin and good looking.

If you want to lose weight to feel better and be healthier and have lower blood sugar, then picture yourself feeling less tired and focus on the things you will be able to do that you are not capable of now.

Visualizing what things will be like during and after your weight loss can be a huge motivation to keep up the effort. Not only that but monitor your progress and make sure you are aware of how much you have progressed.

Maybe you can walk twice as fast or twice as long now as you could when you started. Maybe you fit into a pair of pants that you couldn't button a month ago. Whatever the example might be, realize it and embrace it.

But most of all, YOU need to want to do this and YOU need to understand WHY you want to do this and what benefits you believe you will get out of it. Only then will you stay motivated to keep up the effort and stay committed.

Your Support Team

While there are some things that people must do by themselves in life, losing weight most certainly isn't one of them. There are so many environment factors that either cause or contribute to the problem; it might be close to impossible for someone to lose weight without the help and support of those around them.

We discuss willpower (or lack of) in another chapter but the fact remains that in order to make any kind of change, you have to do something different. Since our brains hate change and will resist it, we have to help our brain along until it is comfortable with the new behavior.

Unless you live alone near no one else and work out of your house, you will be interacting with other people.

These people can either make your progress a lot easier or make it almost impossible. That is why it is important to make the people around you part of your support team.

When you start trying to change what you eat and substitute different food for what you are currently eating, that can become really difficult to keep committed to when those around you are eating junk food and candy and pastries.

For example, if your office is the kind where they bring in all kinds of snacks and pastries and ice cream every day, you will find yourself tempted almost constantly and eventually you will give in and have something you told yourself you wouldn't. Once you do that, the next time is easier and the time after that even easier.

The same goes for home. If your family stocks the pantry and refrigerator with all the foods you love but want to cut back on; that makes it really tempting for you to nibble and snack. The result is that you don't lose any weight. When you are watching TV or even eating a meal and everyone around you is having high calorie snacks while you try to cut back; that can be difficult as well.

While it is not fair to expect others to sacrifice what they eat because someone else wants to lose weight, most people are very willing to make small adjustments to help someone they know.

This is especially true for family members. If Mom or Dad wants to lose weight, most families will plan healthier, lower calorie meals as a substitute for the burgers and fries and milkshakes they usually have on Fridays.

The whole point of this is to get those people around you into your support team. Have a family meeting and tell them what you want to do and why you want to do it. Ask them for their support and assistance. Try and brainstorm ways to make things easier on everyone. Come up with a plan that works for everyone and helps you achieve your goals as well.

The same goes for the office as well. Tell a few close friends or co-workers about your attempt to lose weight. Bring in some low calorie foods or snacks for people to share in the office. The funny thing is the older your co-workers get, the more they restrict their intake of high calorie foods as well. So there might be a little resistance but not a large amount.

Sometimes by just telling people you will find support from others as well. People will say that they have been meaning to lose weight as well and they will join you. Maybe even invite you on a lunchtime walk or exercise class.

Do not attempt to do this all on your own without the help and support of those around you. Most people will support you. The idiot who stands at your door licking a chocolate fudge ice cream cone and moaning can do take a hike. He's just a jerk anyway!

Losing weight is not something you should be embarrassed about. Just the opposite, it should be something you are product to be doing because you want to make your life better and healthier.

So when you're ready, get started building your support team. Not only will they help you achieve your goals, they will provide support for you at the same time. It's something most people really need and everything should really have.

How We Got Here….

Before we get into the real "meat and potatoes" of losing weight, let's pause for a moment to take a look at how we got here. Because knowing how we got to this point is sometimes the most important part of getting to where we want to be.

It seems a lot of people disagree with something I'm going to say right now. At times it seems like society in general disagrees with me but I'm going to say this anyway.

If there is something that needs to be changed, you need to take responsibility for changing what got you here in the first place. If you are not willing to acknowledge how you got here, there is little chance you will get where you want to go!

I'm not particularly big on excuses because excuses do not help you change anything. In fact, they often get in your way.

If you take the position that you did nothing to contribute to where you were, how are you going to convince yourself that you can influence where you want to be?

It sees that today a lot of people do not feel the need to accept responsibility for anything. I have heard stories where overweight people blame restaurants and their huge portions. As if someone forced them to order what they ordered and then not let them leave until they finished it all. Sometimes this just doesn't make sense.

Now sometimes there are issues and conditions that can cause or at least contribute to weight gain. I'm not saying any of that is your fault, not you need to at least recognize it and take responsibility for whatever situation you might find yourself in.

As far as medical conditions are concerned, perhaps this might be an exception. If that is the case, you get a "free pass" on that only if your doctor gives it to you. You do NOT have the right to give it to yourself.

I would also like to make another thing perfectly clear. Accepting responsibility is not the same as accepting blame. This is not about assessing blame or making anyone feel bad. It is all about how you got to where you are today and how we are going to make changes so you can make progress.

It is perfectly fine to look back and see things you did that contributed to your weight loss. You might have had some very good reasons for doing the things that you did. But now, as you look back, if some of those things caused other problems, you do not have to take blame, but you need to accept responsibility for the things that you have done.

As we move forward, I want you to step up and take responsibility for everything that you do. Some things will work out great while others might not go so well. That's OK as long as you accept responsibility for your decisions and actions.

If you eat when you are sad or depressed, just acknowledge it. Don't blame yourself or feel bad about, acknowledge it. If you find yourself eating fast food or garbage food all week long, write it down and acknowledge it. If you are a snack monster and eat a quart of ice cream every night, acknowledge that as well.

Don't make excuses for what you do or ignore it, just acknowledge it. The first step is acknowledging what you do so you can proceed to the next step which is figuring out what to do about it!

You can have all the best reasons for doing what you do. You might look at something you do and find real value in it for you and there is nothing wrong with that. But when it comes to eating, no matter how good a reason you have for eating something, that "something" still has calories in it!

By acknowledging these activities or habits we discover the things that bring us further away from our goals as well as the things that bring us closer to our goals. We can't change everything nor should we try. But the more we acknowledge the things we do the more we understand the option that we have to change things.

A wonderful thing happens when we accept responsibility for our actions. When we accept responsibility for the things that we do we start to care about what we do and how we do it. We make better decisions and we act more decisively when we need to. We empower ourselves to make changes in our lives that help us make things better.

If you tend to overeat when you are sad or stressed, so be it. Accepting responsibility for that response is the first thing that needs to happen before you can change what you do. When we blame others we often fail to take action. When we accept responsibility we also accept the realization that we can control our own destiny.

So please, whatever it is that you might do moving forward, stand up and take responsibility for it. Celebrate your success and learn from your failures. You will gain a wealth of pride and success in the process

The Willpower Myth

One of the most common things I hear from people is that they have no willpower. In other words, they claim they cannot keep themselves focused and committed to anything for long periods of time. They start out with great intentions and a ton of enthusiasm but then it kind of falls apart.

Well, count me in as one of "those people" because I don't have much will power either. Chances are you don't have it either because most people do not have what is commonly called "willpower".

Willpower as we know it and refer to it is a myth. No one can sustain focus and effort and sacrifice over a long period of time. OK, maybe not everybody, but pretty damned close to no one. Most people have a certain limit on how long they can keep up their commitment and focus and concentration.

What follows now is very important because I'm about to make everyone feel just a little bit better about themselves and a lot more confident of what lies ahead for them.

People do NOT achieve success with something because of willpower. Willpower might carry them through the early stages of a task or goal but there is no way most people can sustain the effort through willpower. So if the key to success is not willpower, what is it?

We achieve success by changing things in such a way that we take an existing behavior or attitude and replace it with another one. We use focus and concentration until this replacement behavior becomes a habit and we just do it without thinking. At that point we do not have to rely on willpower or concentration or anything. It just becomes a habit and it happens by itself.

As a basic example, let's say that I love hot fudge sundaes. I mean, I really love them. I have one four or five times a week. But I gain a lot of weight because the damned things have about 1,500 calories in each one!

So instead of having the hot fudge sundaes, I find something else I really like and have that instead of the hot fudge sundaes. Let's say I also love Oreo cookies. So instead of that hot fudge sundae with its 1,500 calories I eat 4 Oreos that have 280 calories for the 4 of them. (OK, I mean I could have said a salad but I'm trying to keep this real!)

The bottom line is that now when you treat yourself 4 or 5 times a week each time you save yourself 1,220 calories or 6,120 calories a week! That would amount to over a pound and a half a week of weight. Just be substituting one treat for another.

When we take one "bad" thing and substitute something "good" or even "less bad" for it we make progress. This is not about sacrifice or eliminating all the good stuff from our diet and starving ourselves. No one can keep starving themselves and denying themselves the things in life they really enjoy for the long term.

We might be able to do it short-term but long term change has to be done with more than just willpower backing it up. So please do not think you are unable to make a meaningful change in your life or your weight because you lack willpower. That kind of attitude is just self-defeating. It is very negative and it is just not true.

Instead, let's move ahead and first determine the things we need to change and then let's figure out how to do it with a minimum amount of focus and concentration. When we are able to do that, we can take all that talk about willpower and toss it right in the trash.

Exactly where it belongs!

Medical Issues & Support

Though this chapter might read as one long disclaimer, the fact is that your family doctor, or specialty doctor if you have one, can be a great ally and resource for you in reaching your weight loss goal safely and in a healthy manner.

In fact, involving your family doctor is not really an option, it is a necessity! Everyone is different and everyone has a certain medical history and physical condition. What is healthy and safe for you might be really dangerous for me or your neighbor. So consult your doctor before starting on any program or activity that is going to change your body in any way.

I think it is very smart to get a physical examination every year. If you are contemplating a weight loss program, why not talk to your doctor while getting that physical. (If you already had one do not put your weight loss off until next year, however!)

If you decide to follow some of the suggestions in this book, bring the book with you and have your doctor look it over and give you their thoughts.

We have made every effort to make the suggestions and activities in this book safe for even the most jaded couch potato but there are medical issues that might have to be considered.

Ask your doctor what is a good start or goal for you. You might think it would be great for you to lose 50 pounds but your doctor might have other ideas. Talk to your doctor and listen to him. Get some blood tests to make certain everything is all right before you start. Everyone should have this done once a year anyway.

One very important thing to watch is blood pressure. Overweight people are more likely to have high blood pressure and that is nothing to ignore or refuse to pay attention to. They do not call it the "silent killer" for nothing! If you have high blood pressure, talk to your doctor about diet and exercise and what you can do and what you can't do. Remember, weight loss is not a race to your goal. It's about getting to your goal in a slow and healthy manner.

Now that you will go to your doctor, the only other thing is something a lot of people do not do when they go to their doctor. That is LISTENING to what he says and recommends. If we go to the doctor but don't follow their suggestions and instructions, then we really can't expect good and healthy results.

Your doctor is not there with the goal of making your life miserable. Instead, they are there to help you live longer and better and keep you healthy.

So when they tell you that you should do something; really try to do it. Just as important, if they tell you that you should NOT do something; really try to not do those things as well. This might mean altering your plan or your goal but your health and life is far more important than an arbitrary deadline.

Listen to your doctor and follow his instructions and guidance! Failure to do so can result in serious medical issues up to and including death!

Do NOT follow what other people did or think that because something worked for someone else it will work and be safe for you!

Losing Weight the Healthy Way

It is important when deciding how to lose weight that we arrive at a plan that is healthy, responsible and achievable. If we fail to include all three of these items in our plan we run the risk of some very unpleasant side effects! With that in mind, here is what we need to do to ensure the best chances of success:

Do Things in a Healthy Manner

There are limitations as far as what we can do to lose weight in a healthy manner. Part of our weight loss plan should include a visit with our family doctor or specialist if one is involved in your health care.

The reason for this is that diet and exercise contribute to changes that occur within your body.

Not only the loss of weight but also internal stress, blood pressure, glucose levels and other items that people like you and I do not have a prayer of understanding. That's why we need our doctors input!

A perfect example of this would be for diabetics who start an exercise or diet program. Since what we eat and how we exercise significantly impacts our blood sugar levels, we need to understand what we need to do to monitor and correct this as we move forward.

For me this meant monitoring my sugars more carefully and eventually cutting back on my medications (that's a great benefit!) to avoid the lows I started getting as I exercised and ate better. By talking with my doctor BEFORE I started, she made me aware of what could happen and how to deal with it. So when I did start to get those lows, I didn't freak out, I just altered my medications.

People with heart issues should always consult with their doctors because diet and exercise can have a HUGE impact on our hearts. We might have to start more slowly and proceed more slowly so we do not overburden our hearts.

We could go on and on with specific health issues and diseases but we will mention just one more. People with high blood pressure should be very careful when it comes to exercise. Most exercise will tend to elevate your blood pressure because we are working our bodies harder.

But if your pressure is already very high, exercise might have to be extremely limited. Again, we need to involve our doctors in our care and weight loss program.

Weight loss is not a race to the end. It is a process that needs to happen in a healthy manner to be effective I both the short and long-term. Crash diets and other weight loss fads might produce quick weight loss but when we do those types of things the weight usually comes back on and then some.

Which brings us to our next focus point.

Act Responsibly

Hey, you can lose weight fast if you eat nothing but a bowl of lettuce and water while you run 15 miles every morning before work. But that is not realistic or responsible.

We have to be responsible when it comes to understanding what the right way is for each of us to lose weight. We need to know ourselves and our eating habits and our own lifestyle. In other words, it is not important to lose weight fast as it is to lose weight in a responsible manner. We want to be successful not be dangerous or unhealthy in our actions.

Being responsible is knowing what we can or can't do and what is the right way for us to proceed. We need to know and understand our limitations and what we are capable of.

For example, we should not design a plan that we know we cannot keep up with. We should not make the sacrifice so high that we know we will give up in a short time. We should know what we can do and what will be too much and then be able to design a plan we can follow and stay on. I have said this once and I will say it again, this is NOT a race. This is a process and we need to give it the time it needs to be successful. Be honest with yourself and design a plan that you can stick to.

Create a Plan that is Achievable

How many things have you started and been excited about only to lose interest and stop after a few days or weeks? If you are like most people, this happens to you a lot of the course of your life.

When people start things they are excited and motivated and fully engaged. They dive right in and are willing to work hard and sacrifice like crazy to achieve their goals. Then, a short time later they say "Screw this! It's just too much work!" Then they give up and go back to what they were doing before.

This does not happen just with weight loss but in any activity that requires work and/or dedication. If we design a plan that is too difficult or requires too much effort, we are drastically reducing our chances for success.

We need to be honest with ourselves when we are designing a weight loss plan. We need to acknowledge our weaknesses and limitations. Sometimes this is not easy but it's something that needs to be done.

As far as acknowledging our weakness and shortcomings are concerned, one thing we cannot do is use these as an excuse. If you don't want to exercise, don't tell yourself you can't because it is a weakness of yours. Weaknesses and shortcomings are a reality but they are not an excuse. We acknowledge them and we work around them when designing our plan. So if you thought you found a way out, think again!

Creating a Plan that is Achievable means coming up with something that you can do that will help you achieve your goal but will not be so difficult that you would give up. It would be a better plan to take 20 weeks of slow and gradual diet and exercise to reach a goal than it would to have a difficult 10 week plan that you would likely give up.

Start off slow and see how you react to your new plan. If it is too much, consider reassessing your plan and make some changes to it. Plans are not cast in stone. They are evolving works in progress. Just design something you can stick with and modify it as you go along.

Your Starting Point

Before you get started, you need to know where you are now. By that I mean what kind of physical condition you are currently in. this will help you design your plan and figure out your exercise levels and other information.

Not everyone is in the same physical condition. Even two people of the same weight can be in totally different physical condition. Add to that diseases or medical issues a person might have and you can really get a wide range of physical conditions.

Lifestyle plays a huge role in this as well. Some people have jobs where they are on their feet all days long while others stay at their desks in a chair all day long. So you can't treat one person like the other and vice versa.

If you haven't talked to your doctor yet, this would be a good time to do so. Even people who feel great and look great might have a really valid reason to take it easy when starting an exercise or diet program.

Go to the expert and get their opinion. They will help you figure out the very best starting point.

You should also start by identifying the level of exercise you are capable of doing at this very moment. Can you walk comfortably for 10 minutes? 20 minutes? 30 minutes? That can give you an idea of where you are as well. Whatever exercise you think you might be doing, see what you can do comfortably right now. That will be your starting point and you will build on that.

Do not worry about what your spouse or neighbor can do. You are you, not them. Let them do what they can do and you do what you should do. Again, this is not a race, it is a journey. We should not rush it but make the journey as pleasant as possible.

It is important throughout this entire process that you be as honest with yourself as possible. If something is honestly too difficult for you, dial things back a bit. But don't do it just so things are easy. Do it because you can't do something not because you don't want to.

The other thing you should be doing is logging what you eat every day. Get a note book and write down everything you eat of the next week or two. Don't change anything or look at it until you have finished the entire week or two that you want to measure.

After you are done, take a look at what you consume every day. You will likely be surprised because little snacks and things add up over the course of a day.

If you want to, buy yourself a calorie book that lists the calories in all kinds of foods and figure out how many calories you consume over the course of a day or week.

I think your will be very surprised.

But all this is good because in order to get where we are going, we have to know where we've been and where we are now.

It is also important to remember that we got to this point in life because of the things we have done up to this point. If we are overweight, it is either because of a medical reason or because we ate too much or exercised too little. It might even be a combination of the three. What matters is that we understand where we are and how we got there. This allows us to target the cause of problem and not waste time fixing something that isn't broken.

Please don't ignore this step and think that you know everything about yourself. It is worth the time to look at your life and actually see what you do, how you do it, and get some insight into why things are the way they are.

This isn't about blame and it isn't about making anyone feel bad. You don't have to share what you discover with anyone. This is for your eyes and ears only. So be honest and truthful with yourself.

Any journey has a beginning, an end, and many steps along the way. It just makes sense to know each and every one of them.

Calories- In & Out

Sometimes I hate calories. I mean whenever I see something that looks really good and then I see how many calories are in it, I hate those calories! But calories are what we need to know in order to make intelligent decisions. So, in that regard, calories are a good thing!

While it is good to know how many calories are in your favorite foods, the most important thing to remember is that 3,500 calories is a rough equivalent to gaining one pound. So, if you eat 3,500 more calories than you burn off in a day, you will gain one pound.

It makes no difference if you ate 3,500 calories of salad, or soup or beef or a hot fudge sundae. If you eat 3,500 more calories of ANYTHING than you burn off, you will gain a pound. So don't think it is all right to eat more of something because it is healthy. A calorie is a calorie is a calorie.

We should mention that NUTRICIANALLY, it makes a big difference because 3,500 calories of vegetables is a lot better than 3,500 calories of chocolate cake! But still calories are calories and we need to be aware of what we eat.

Now the coolest thing is that we can eat whatever we want if we can burn those calories off! That's right! If we can burn those extra calories off, we can have the foods we love and not gain weight!

It's really a very simple concept. We can eat whatever we want as long as we burn up the calories we eat. Whether we eat chocolate cake, hot fudge sundaes or our other favorite foods we can eat them as long as we burn those calories during the day!

How do we burn those calories? Well our metabolism, which we will cover in another chapter, will cause us to burn off calories as we go through our day. Every step we take, every movement we make, and time we take a breath, we expend energy and burn calories. The more we do, the more calories we burn!

The average number of calories we burn every day to just sustain life and do our basic activities without scheduled exercise is roughly 10 calories per pound of body weight if you are a woman and 11 calories per pound if you are a man. So if you are a 200 pound man you would burn approx 200 X 11 or 2200 calories per day. If you are a 150 pound woman that would be 150 X 10 or 1500 calories a day.

To that total you would add any calories burned by any type of exercise you would do during the day. That would include scheduled exercise plus other activities such as mowing the lawn, cleaning the house, even cooking can burn up calories!

These are just basic numbers and your actual number depends on your own metabolism and body. You might burn more or less in an average day. If you are a couch potato and move very little during the day it would be lower. If you are somewhat active, you would burn more, if you are very active, you would burn even more!

So the first step would be to take our list of foods that we eat during an average day and add up the calories using either our calorie book of reading the food labels. This will give us the approximate number of calories we consume each day.

This is why it is so important to be as accurate and honest as possible when writing down your food list and portion size. If you skip some items or write down smaller portions because you don't want people to know what you eat you are only cheating yourself. No one other than you needs to see this list so make it accurate and make it honest and complete. That is the only way to give yourself the best chance of success!

Now, if you discover you are eating 2,000 calories a day and you are a 190 pound man, you are close to being on track as your approx calories burned would be 190 X 11 or 2090 per day.

But even those 90 extra calories would add up at the end of the year! 90 extra calories a day for 365 days would come to 32,850 calories. That would be equal to gaining 9.38 pounds a year! (32,850 divided by 3,500 calories per pound)

Since just 90 calories a day (less than a chocolate bar) can add up to a lot of weight at the end of the year, we want to be very careful to stay at or lower the number of calories we burn. No one ever complained about having to eat more on occasion because they were losing weight. But the gradual addition of weight can be frustrating.

Now if you find that you are eating 3,500 calories a day, you have some tough decisions ahead of you because you need to do something significant to burn off those extra calories. 3,500 calories a day is a LOT of calories but you would be shocked to see how quickly those calories can add up. A fast food lunch can be 2,000 calories right there. Add to that a couple of donuts and a latte for breakfast and some steak and French fries for dinner and you're at 3,500 before those late night snacks!

We will get into this more in other chapters but it is important to understand where your calories are coming from. Sometimes just by being aware you can cut the number of calories significantly without sacrifice! For example, for years when I went to the ballpark I would buy the tub of popcorn. After all popcorn is the "healthy" snack and the tub would last all ballgame.

But then they started putting the calories on the signs and I almost had a heart attack right there because the popcorn had 2,700 calories. I could have eaten 5 hotdogs and saved 100 calories! Even sugary cotton candy only had 300 calories!

Weight loss is not about telling yourself you can't eat the food you love. It IS all about telling yourself to be aware of what you eat and how many calories you consume. Knowledge is power and knowing what you are eating, and the calories in those foods, enables you to make decisions that will make weight loss easier and more successful without a ton of sacrifice!

So if you have not started your food journal yet, start one now. If you have not purchased a calorie book, or downloaded one online, do that now as well. Then started learning how many calories you consume!

Get Ready, Get Set, SWITCH!

The best way to start losing weight is by getting rid of some of those high calorie foods. Not necessarily eliminating them totally, but getting them out of our daily diet. Sometimes this is not easy because taking away the food we love is not something that is a positive experience. But there are things we can do to make this process a lot easier.

First, we always come back to this but know your body and know what you need to do and what it is going to take to get you there. This is important because we need to understand what amount of change is going to need to happen for us to reach our goals.

For example, if we discover that we are eating 300 calories a day more than what we need to eat in order to lose weight, we need to trim at least 300 calories a day to start.

We can do that with a few minor changes that will be easy to make. This will make our chances of success far greater and we will be more likely to stay on track for a longer period of time.

But if we are eating 800 calories more a day than we need, then eliminating 300 is a move in the right direction but we will still be gaining weight! So we need to change even more to get those 800 extra calories eliminated.

Our best chances of success are not eliminating things. Eliminating something only works when we replace it with something that fits our plan a lot better.

Eliminating something means sacrifice and we don't like sacrifice. So we will have a much better chance of success if we substitute those foods with something else. The result is that we lower calorie count while still eating the right amount of food.

For example, if you are having a big bowl of ice cream with chocolate sauce on it every night, that adds thousands of calories a week on to your calorie intake. But if we can find something else you like, such as some fruit or Jell-O, you could reduce calories while still having something you enjoy as your snack. This way you are not sacrificing your enjoyment you are just substituting one snack for another.

Another example might be salad dressing. Do not give up dressing on your salads but substitute a low fat or reduced calorie dressing instead. A little change like this can add up at the end of the week.

Perhaps the biggest change can be made in what you drink. Every can of soda is between 140 and 180 calories. If you drink 2 cans a day, that's 14 cans a week or 1960 – 2520 calories per week.

If you can find a diet soda that you enjoy, you would save 101,920 – 131,040 calories a year. That equates to approx. 29 – 37 POUNDS of weight loss just by switching to a diet soda! Even switching just half the time, one can per day, could mean a weight loss of 14-18 pounds a year!

Think about your soda consumption, all those high fat lattes and hot chocolates and yes, your alcohol consumption. Alcohol has a ton of calories in it and those can really add up. The term "beer belly" does not come from people who are skinny beer drinkers! Again, this is all about being aware of what you are eating and making small changes that could give you big results!

We are not asking you to eliminate all the things you like, just find something to substitute for the high calorie foods. Which do you think might be easier for you: giving up the big bowl of ice cream with chocolate syrup and having nothing as a mid night snack or substituting the ice cream with some Jell-O with whipped cream? Or, if you are intent on the ice cream maybe, just maybe, we could switch to some low fat and lower calorie ice cream?

Many of us just have to make some minor changes to get the weight to start coming off. The whole idea is to find the point where you start to lose weight and then keep things going at that pace.

This is how you keep weight off for years.

Most people go on drastic diets and eliminate all the foods they like and they sacrifice everything. They sweat and fret and struggle through until they lost the weight they wanted to.

Then they go back to what they were doing before and the weight comes back on. Usually these people put back on MORE weight when they go back to their original eating habits.

By substituting foods and behaviors, we create a new way of behaving and eating that will not only help us take the weight off, but keep it off in the long run.

Sacrifice

I don't really like sacrifice and I assume you don't either. Doing without something you love or like is not a pleasant process and we should do without it as long as possible. But we also need to be responsible human beings and take care of our health. So it's kind of a balancing act and one that we need to address.

As we have stated, losing weight means that we have to alter some of our behaviors. Sometimes this entails sacrifice other times it doesn't. Our goal should be to accomplish our intended goal with as little sacrifice as possible.

There is nothing wrong with not wanting to sacrifice. It is not selfish or irresponsible. Rather it might be construed as being smart. Think about one thing for a moment.

What would you be more likely to do; something that is hard and requires a ton of sacrifice or something that was easier and required much less sacrifice?

If we are really being honest, almost everyone would choose the easy road with little sacrifice. Even if it takes more time, people are willing to take a little more time to minimize sacrifice.

At some point we are going to have decisions to make. We will need to choose between time and sacrifice or between more than one option. Would we rather sacrifice eating a particular food or would we rather exercise a bit more and eat that food? Weight loss is not a black and white process. We can accomplish the same goals in more than one way. We just have to understand our options, understand ourselves, and make the right choices.

Sacrifice can be limited, possibly even eliminated if we have the knowledge that enables us to make informed decisions. Sacrifice can be controlled when we know what needs to be done and what the best ways are to get those things done.

Sacrifice can be minimized when we understand what is happening and why it is happening. After all, why should do we take the hard road when the easier path will bring us to the same destination?

There are those people who say that hard work is necessary in order to achieve anything of value. I respectfully disagree. I say that it is better to work smart than work hard. If you can use information and knowledge to make things easier and increase your chances for success then you should use it!

The fact is, the easier we make a task the more likely it is that we will stick with it. The easier something is the more people will attempt it and achieve success.

Again, for the umpteenth time, weight loss is not a race but a process. If we make that process easier and less stressful, the greater our chances of success will be.

So let's target our efforts on becoming successful and not consume ourselves with sacrifice. We don't have to do this but that's not something I am willing to sacrifice!

Setting Up for Success!

Most of us are creatures of habit and we will tend to continue doing the things we have been doing until we are forced to do otherwise. We talked about the myth of willpower and how we cannot depend on sheer focus and determination for long term success. It is just too much effort and requires too much dedication. In order to achieve long-term success we need to make adjustments to our lifestyle. That also includes our environment.

Our environment is one of the largest factors in our ability, or inability, to lose weight. The places and things around us have a profound impact on what we eat, when we eat it, and how often we eat. In order to lose weight, we need to take a strong look at our environment.

We all have our weaknesses and we need to do something to help us get over those weaknesses.

The biggest factor when it comes to what we eat is convenience. If something is very convenient to us, we will tend to take advantage of that and food is no different. If it's there, we will most likely eat it!

With that in mind, take a few moments to rid yourself of the foods that you really don't want to eat anymore. I'm not saying to throw food away. Maybe donate it to a food pantry or bring it in to work for a Friday feast or something but just get it out of your house.

If there are others in your household and they have food around that tempts you, perhaps they would be willing to store that food in their room or hide it away someplace where it is out of your mind. You can't expect others to diet or give up what they like just because you don't want to eat it but they can help you.

Do the same thing at work. Remove the hidden food in your desk drawers and the stuff in the break room refrigerator with your name on it. If you don't have it nearby, you won't be as likely to eat it.

The important thing to remember is that most cravings are short term events. If you get a craving for some Oreos, that craving will only last a short time. If you have Oreos in the house, you will be tempted to eat them. But if you have to get dressed, get in the car, drive to the supermarket and buy some, then drive home, that's most often enough time for the craving to pass. Most of the time the sheer effort involved is enough to discourage us from giving in to the craving.

As you can hopefully see, we are taking steps to eliminate willpower from the equation and instead rely on other factors. By ridding our homes and other areas of the foods we decide we no longer want to eat, we eliminate willpower and substitute inconvenience to help us stay away from those foods.

Think about how many times you walked by the pantry and grabbed a handful of chips, or M&M's or a few cookies. Over the course of the day there little indulgences can add up to 1,000 calories a day or more! Heck, just two Oreos will set you back 100 calories! Same with a handful of chips! It does not take much to pile on a ton of extra calories over the course of a day!

Not having these foods around just makes it easier to avoid the temptation. It does NOT mean you can never eat them. If you really want the Oreo's, then go out to the store and buy a small package and have them. We should not be worried about the occasional couple of cookies. It is when we have those two cookies 10 times a day and are constantly snacking that can do us in.

Impulse snacking is dangerous because we do it almost without thinking. We grab something here, snack on something there and never really think about all the calories we are consuming. When we have to make a conscious effort to go out and buy something, we have a lot of time to think about what we are going to eat and how many calories are involved. Often times this will make us think twice and stop right there.

That is what we are trying to accomplish with creating an environment that helps you towards your goals not one that keeps you from those goals.

So let's go through that pantry, refrigerator, freezer and everywhere else you store your food and do a spring cleaning. Get rid of the stuff you do not want to eat anymore. Help yourself lose weight by creating the proper environment. It is a process that will work very well for you if you give it half a chance!

Negative Calorie Foods

Here is an interesting concept. Negative calorie foods are foods that require more energy and calories to digest than they actually have in them. What that means is that you burn more calories during the processing and digesting of those foods than they had in the food itself.

Here is a list of some negative calorie foods:

Fruits

Apples
Cranberries
Grapefruit
Lemon
Mango
Orange
Pineapple
Raspberries
Strawberries
Tangerine
Vegetables

Asparagus
Beets
Brocoli
Cabbage
Carrots
Cauliflower
Celery
Chili peppers (hot)
Cucumber
Dandelion
Endive
Garden cress
Garlic
Green beans
Lettuce
Onion
Papaya
Radishes
Spinach

We are not saying to create an entire diet made up of these fruits and vegetable but it certainly couldn't hurt to use some of these items in your meals and snacks. Not only will you fill yourself up, but they are essentially "free" calories when used in moderation.

If you want a more complete listing of these foods, or some more information on negative calorie foods, just go online and do a search under "negative calorie foods".

Just make sure they are part of a balanced and nutritious diet and do not over do it!

Exercise!

AAAAHHHH! There it is! The dirty word all weight loss plans include that frightens the hearts of most of us! But, hey, calm down for a moment. This is not going to be as hard as you think it is. In fact, you just might be a little bit relieved!

When people think of exercise, they usually think about sweating, running marathons and endless working out at the gym. Though exercise can take those forms it is also important that exercise can take other forms that are a lot less intense and still beneficial to us as far as our health and losing weight.

Regardless of the type of exercise you choose, all exercise has one thing I common. Exercise burns calories. The more intense and active the exercise might be, the more calories you will burn in an hour.

A long distance runner and a person bowling are both burning calories but the runner is burning more per hour than the bowler.

But the bottom line here is that it is not so much how many calories we are burning but how long we exercise and making sure we burn more calories each day than we are taking in!

Someone once told me they didn't feel that they were accomplishing very much. They were older and not capable of doing much exercise. They figured they were only burning off an extra 100 calories a day. When I told them that still was 36,500 or 10 pounds of weight, they were shocked!

So ask yourself which is better, doing a little bit of exercise and burning off 100 calories or doing nothing and burning off 10 calories. Every little bit adds up and no exercise is too little.

Experts say that to get the most benefit from any kind of exercise you need to do it for between 24 minutes and 60 minutes. This is not so much for weight loss but for cardiac fitness. Once you get past 24 minutes you start reaping cardio vascular benefits which is a bonus for you.

But the fact is that ANY exercise you get is better than no exercise at all. It is better to start slow than not start at all. Even if you can only manage to walk for 5 minutes, walk those 5 minutes. Then make it 6 minutes, then 7, then 10, whatever you become capable of. This is not a race, it is a journey. Never lose sight of that!

When it comes to the type of exercise; that should be left up to personal preference. Pick a sport you like so exercise becomes fun. Make it a social event as well by joining a bowling league or tennis club.

Anything you can do to make it more tolerable or enjoyable will help you stick with it.

Even activities such as landscaping or mowing the lawn will burn off some calories. Anything that gets you up and constantly moving will help you burn calories and get in better shape. The key is doing something you enjoy. Remember, nothing is too little to start. Taking it slow and gradually building yourself up is the way to go. Doing it slowly and do it safely and you will get to where you want to go.

One of the easiest forms of exercise for anyone of any age is walking. We will be using that as our way of getting some exercise without a great deal of sweating. Walking is something most of us can do even if only for short periods of time.

Walking Off the Weight

Walking is a form of exercise that is very convenient and very easy on the muscles and bones. Almost everyone can do it and even people in wheelchairs can push themselves around the block or the mall and burn some calories. I happen to enjoy walking for a few important reasons.

Walking is something that can be done at just about any fitness level. Those of us not in very good condition can start off very slow until we are able to go faster. There is no embarrassment and very little chance of injury unless you misstep and fall or twist an ankle.

Walking can be done just about anywhere. You can do it outside on a nice day or go inside at the mall or supermarket when it is raining or a little too cold for you. Malls are great because you can get distracted by looking at the people and the windows in the shops and walk more than you originally thought! Plus, malls are heated and air conditioned so you won't have to worry about being too hot or too cold.

I have taken to adding exercise into my grocery shopping. I will get an item, then walk around the perimeter of the store, get my second item, walk around the perimeter and so on. You would be surprised how many extra steps and distance you can add doing this!

If you have a treadmill, that's even better because you can start off really, really slow and build up distance and speed over time moving ahead only when you feel ready. If you are able, you can even add running into parts of your walk to get the cardio benefits and increase the number of calories burned every hour.

Before starting any exercise you should check with your doctor to see if it is advisable and at what level you should start. Follow their directions as they know your body better than anyone.

For those of you who won't check with your doctor, an accepted gauge of exertion is that if you can carry on a normal conversation with someone while you are exercising, that is a good pace. If you are huffing and puffing and can't talk, you are pushing too hard.

Another universal kind of goal is that everyone does 10,000 steps a day. That's a good number of steps and most of us will have to increase our activity level to hit that. But it is very achievable for just about anyone.

Speaking of steps, I strongly urge anyone who wants to lose weight to go out and purchase a pedometer. A pedometer is a device that counts the steps we take during the day. They are not expensive and a good one will cost you less than $20. Maybe even $10 if you find one on sale.

There are two types of pedometers. One has a mechanical mechanism that has a pendulum inside that swings during every step. These are not that accurate especially for heavier people with considerable fat around the waist. That is because this type of pedometer has to be pretty much straight up and down and heavier people usually have their belts tilted down. For me personally, I used a pendulum model until I compared it to a better one and found I was only getting credit for half my steps!

The other models use something called an accelerometer. This is an electronic sensor which measures movement. These are far more accurate and these are not that expensive either. Check online and on EBAY or Amazon for the best deals.

One word of caution for the accelerometer models, however. They tend to give you steps while riding in a car or motorcycle. That is because they sense movement. So you will have to take a reading before getting in the car and read it again when you get out.

Subtract the number of steps added during the car trip and you will have an accurate daily reading.

The pedometer is a great tool because it lets you know how you are doing during the day. If you only have 1,000 steps by lunchtime, you might take a walk or do something to get a little more active. Making small corrections to increase your walking earlier in the day helps avoid having to take a big walk at night!

A pedometer also helps you discover "hidden" activities that burn off more calories than you might think. For example, I was surprised to see I had taken 2,000 steps doing grocery shopping. And that was before I did that "walking the perimeter" thing! I am a strong believer in building your exercise into your daily routine so you get it without realizing it.

Little changes can really add up. For example parking at the end of the parking lot and walking further to work can easily add 500 steps to your day. Taking a walk during a break or lunch can rack up steps too! Mowing my lawn is good for 3,000 steps! Every little bit helps.

I am a strong believer in the 10,000 steps a day goal. It is small enough that most people can hit the goal without too much trouble.

But if you can't why not make it a 5,000 step goal? Or, let's talk about doing something custom for your own weight loss plan.

Get yourself a pedometer and see how much you normally walk each day. Measure this over a full week.

Then divide the total steps by 7 days to get your average. Add 10 percent to that and make that your new daily goal. When that gets easy for you, add another 10% and so on until you get to where you want to be.

That is why walking is so great. You can do it fast or slow, for as long or short a distance as you feel you are up to. Go around the block or walk around town. Whatever fitness level you currently are at walking can easily help you out.

Walking is also great for people who are in very poor condition. Some people have a hard time doing any sports or physical exercise. But unless there is a disability or medical reason involved, they can still walk. Even if it is just once around the backyard, keep doing that. Then maybe one and a half times, then two times. Eventually around the block. Take it as slow as you need to. Do not rush it or push too hard.

This is all about finding the right level of exercise for you. A level that will enable you to get exercise but still keep at it for the long-term. There is no need to push yourself to the point where you feel bad or sick or until you are wringing wet with sweat. If that is what you want to do, that's fine. But it is not what you NEED to do.

We want to figure out some form of exercise that we can keep doing every week for the foreseeable future. Losing weight and keeping ourselves fit and healthy is not a one month or one year process. It is all about changing how we live our lives.

But this doesn't mean we have to take away the things we love and substitute things we hate. Rather it means being smart and figuring out how to get as much of what we want and need as possible.

I found out in the last year how just one hour of exercise 3 days a week could make my blood sugar levels go down so much that I had to reduce my medicine. I found out that one hour a day, three days a week was not hard and the benefits were amazing. I had more energy. I wasn't as tired as I used to be and I could do more than I could 2 or 3 years ago!

This is not some kind of magic pills or fantasy. It is a great way to make a huge difference in the quality of life that you have now and in your future. I urge you find something, anything, to get you off the couch and become more active. Every little bit counts, every little bit helps, and every little bit brings you closer to your goals and dreams.

Anyone care to go for a walk?

Metabolism

While this is not a medical based program or publication, we still would like to discuss something that has a very critical role in whether we lose weight or how fast we lose weight. That factor is our metabolism.

Metabolism is the activity that goes on inside our cells that allows them to survive and for us to live. It is the process our bodies use to convert calories into energy. One of the influences this has on our bodies is to influence how fast or slow our bodies burn calories. If you have a very high metabolism, you will likely be thinner as you burn more calories per hour 24 hours a day than someone with a low metabolism.

Our metabolism is mostly due to genetics but there are a few things we can do to "speed it up" and increase the amount of calories we burn in a day.

If we are able to make our metabolism higher, we will lose weight faster and tend to keep it off longer.

At this point I must caution you that our metabolism is critical for our overall health. Do not go crazy and try all sorts of things to make it higher and higher. As with everything, moderation and health are the keys to success.

Our metabolism is also affected by our body weight and composition. The more lean muscle we have the higher our metabolism becomes. Conversely, if we have a lot of fat on our body, that will slow down our metabolism.

Another factor, and this is unfair, is that as we age, our metabolism usually slows down. This is just part of aging and one of the reasons our bodies change shape and composition over time. The older we get, the more we have to do to keep our bodies the same. As I said, that seems unfair!

There are a few things we can do to increase our metabolism. The great thing is that these are the very things we also need to do to lose weight. So every time you do these things, you accomplish two things at the same time. You lose weight and you increase your metabolism which in turn helps you lose weight even more!

Here are a few things you can do to increase your metabolism:

Exercise more often – Exercise builds lean muscle. Muscles burn more calories than weight pound for pound so the more muscle you have the more calories you will burn!

Get Cardio exercise – Cardio exercise burns more calories per hour than regular exercise and the benefits to the body are many.

One of the great benefits of cardio exercise is that the calorie burning caused by the exercise continues for about an hour after you stop exercising! So you burn even more calories than you thought!

Build muscle – Muscle burns more calories than fat and muscle helps you exercise longer and more often and makes it easier to do the things you need to in life. The more muscle on your frame, the higher your metabolism.

Don't skip meals! – One of the things a lot of people do is skip meals because they believe they will save calories and increase weight loss. The fact is skipping meals can do the opposite because when you starve your body it reacts by slowing down your metabolism in order to conserve energy. Your best approach is to eat every meal as scheduled but just be careful with what you eat. If you are a diabetic, skipping meals can lead to wild variations in glucose levels which is not good for the body.

Eat protein – Protein usually requires more calories to digest and also gives you body the nutrients it needs to function properly.

Eat breakfast – some consider breakfast the most important meal of the day. Eating a good and healthy breakfast gets your metabolism going and helps you burn more calories during the day. In case you are wondering, a cup of coffee does not qualify as a healthy breakfast!

Get moving – If you do a lot of sitting during the day that will tend to slow down your metabolism. Get up and stretch, move around and be more active. Not only will this burn more calories, it will keep your metabolism from going to sleep with the rest of you!

Get some sleep – Sleep is very important as that is when the body takes time to heal and refresh itself. If you do not get enough sleep, your metabolism will suffer. Also, your muscles use sleep time to recover from your latest exercise and prepare themselves for the next day. Getting less sleep than you need is counterproductive.

Eat right – a healthy diet that is not rich in fat and sugars will not only help your metabolism but also will help your overall health and also assist you in losing weight. Eliminate as many of those "empty calories" as possible for higher metabolism and better overall health!

Again, we need to say that we are not doctors or medical experts. The information is this chapter is designed only to make you aware of your metabolism and easy things that you can do to help you in your weight loss program. We strongly urge you to talk to a medical professional to get more information on your particular situation so you can do what is best for you.

Medical help will make the entire process easier, more efficient, and safer for you in the long run.

We have said it before and we will say it again; Make your doctor part of your weight loss program.

Another factor concerning your metabolism could be any medical issues or diseases that you might have that influence metabolism. Everyone is different and only your doctor can properly advise you.

Using Metabolism to Help You Lose Weight

Think of your metabolism as a tool to help you get the most out of your weight loss efforts. I know people say there is nothing wrong with hard work and they are correct. But if there was something you could do that would make something easier, wouldn't you be a fool not to take advantage of it?

By doing the little things you need to boost your metabolism, you will create a calorie burning system within your body that will help you burn more calories 24 hours a day without any additional effort on your part!

To lose weight we have to consume fewer calories than we burn so we have a choice to make. We can either eat less of the foods we like, we can exercise even more, or we can create a fat burning metabolism that will help us accomplish the same thing easier.

All of the information you have been reading has been designed not to accomplish magical things for you. It has been designed to make you AWARE. When you are aware of something that can help you, you are more inclined to take advantage of it.

Metabolism is something you should be very aware of. It can make your weight loss process easier and faster and help you continue to keep that weight off after you have hit your goal.

Making Changes
(Moderation)

All right, we are all excited and ready to get started on our journey to lose some weight. I say "journey" to remind you that this is not a race. Unless there is some special reason why you have to accomplish this process as quickly as possible (medical reasons?), you should not view this as something you need to rush through. In the case of weight loss, slow and sure is a lot better than fast and reckless.

Whenever we start on a weight loss program we need to understand a few basic things as to how this weight loss is going to affect our bodies.

First of all, there will be some chemical changes going on as we eat less, exercise more and turn from storing fat to burning fat.

While these changes themselves present little to be concerned about, we go not want to shock the body too much in the process. For that reason, if we are planning major changes in our diet, it might be best to implement them gradually over time.

Remember that our body treats a reduction in eating with a slowing down of the metabolism. In order to stop that from happening, do not suddenly eat far less than you normally would. Gradually reduce your diet to avoid this from happening.

Second, when we exercise we will be using muscles we didn't normally use and some of them will not be thrilled with the process. They will let you know in the form of soreness and aches until they get used to what we are doing. If we try to do too much, too soon, those aches can turn into pulls or worse.

Exercise should be gradually introduced at a rate that is both comfortable but productive. Start slowly and gradually increase the duration and intensity of your workouts so your body can adjust itself. Over time your muscles will strengthen and grow and allow you to do more. But in the beginning, when some of them are waking up from years of hibernation, they cannot handle sudden increases in use.

It is also worth mentioning that you might feel perfectly fine doing something in the beginning but the soreness and other issues will not show up until the next day or so. So don't think because you feel fine now that it is OK to walk those 34 miles the first day out!

Now is also a great time to repeat something for the 35th time! Get your doctor involved in your weight loss program. Let them guide you on how much you should eat and how long you should exercise. They know best what's right for you!

There is another reason why doing everything in moderation is so important. As we said before, our bodies and our brains dislike change. They want everything to go along the same way forever. So when we introduce any kind of change, sometimes our bodies and mind rebel.

If we hit ourselves with massive dietary changes and huge amounts of exercise all at once, this can overload our brains and they will do their best to get us to stop whatever we are doing and go back to the way things used to be. They will use every trick they can to get you to do that. They will make you hurt, feel hungry, give you craving, make you feel overwhelmed and all other kinds of goodies.

So let's stop that nonsense before it begins. Do everything in moderation. That includes dietary changes and exercise. Work new changes in over days and weeks. Start small and work your way up until you are where you need to be. We are going to repeat ourselves because this is so important. Losing weight is NOT a race. It should be done carefully and slowly over time.

Your plan should be to lose no more than 1 or 2 pounds a week.

Even that might become too ambitious after a while. 2 pounds in the first few weeks might be doable but when things slow down, 1 pound might be more reasonable.

Do NOT create a starvation diet to get rapid weight loss. This does NOT work for the long-term. No one can sustain a starvation diet for long without suffering health issues due to the diet! Reduce your caloric intake but do it responsibly and gradually for the best and longest lasting results.

When it comes to exercise, find your comfortable starting point and slowly build from there. When it comes to walking, which is the best way to start any exercise program, find a comfortable starting distance and do that every other day for a week. Then increase the distance the next week no more than 10% that will allow your muscles to grow and heal properly.

Any time we make things harder than we need to we greatly increase our chances of failure. We are much more likely to keep up the effort when our brains say to us "Hey, that's not so bad. I can do this!" If we can get to that point we have the battle half won.

The whole purpose is to make the entire process as easy as possible on our bodies and our mind. Doing something that is easier and less stressful is always good. It might take a little bit longer but ultimately you will have better results and a greater chance of losing the weight you wanted to lose.

Labels

One of your best friends when it comes to losing weight is the nutrition labels that come on food packages. Not only will they help you with counting or measuring calories, they will also help you choose lower fat foods and make other dietary choices.

These labels are on all types of foods but you have to be careful how you read them. There are no "standard" serving sizes so one package might say it has 100 calories a serving but the serving size is 1 ounce. Another package might say it has 200 calories per serving but their serving size is 4 ounces! So the package with the higher calories per serving actually has fewer calories in it! ALWAYS compare serving sizes when looking at labels!

Other useful listings on the labels are grams of carbohydrates and sugar content both of which are very important to diabetics.

Diabetics need to keep their intake of carbs and sugars down and labels help them accomplish that a lot more easily.

One such important item on the label is sodium (salt). Foods that are high in sodium will cause you to drink more fluids and retain more water. So if you eat a high sodium meal, you may find yourself weighing more the next day. This might be just water weight which will disappear over the next day or so. But it also might be because you were thirsty and had 4 cans of non diet soda after the meal which will add a lot of calories to your daily intake. Sodium should also be limited in people who have high blood pressure as well. So just try and stay away from high sodium food and also limit the amount of salt you add to your foods during preparation and meals.

While labels are great, they do not help us when we go out to dinner. But if we eat at certain restaurants, they may have a calorie sheet for their patrons. Depending on where you live, it might even be a law that calories have to be displayed on menus and overhead ordering signage.

If you are a fast food lover, there is good news in that almost every fast food chain has a nutrition listing that lists calories and fat content and a lot of other things about each of their foods. You can use this listing to make your food choices to keep calories and fat levels down.

We stress knowledge a lot in this book because knowledge is what allows us to make informed and accurate decisions. When we refer to these nutrition labels we can pick lower calorie foods that sometime surprise us when it comes to calories.

For example, it is almost a universal belief that chicken is lower in fat and calories and better for you than beef.

But if you walk into a fast food place and order the chicken sandwich, it usually has a lot MORE calories in it than the burgers! As we mentioned in another part of this book, when we went to the ball park their pop corn had more calories than 5 hotdogs!!! And popcorn is supposed to be a healthy snack! Often it is not so much what you are eating but how it is prepared. Sauces, oils and other ingredients can send calorie and fat content soaring!

The key here is to make intelligent choices. Sometimes by looking at labels we can find that a different brand of a certain food has fewer calories. When we find this we can lower calorie count without sacrifice! As we say over and over, it doesn't have to hurt to accomplish something if you can find a better way!

Just think of these labels and menu sheets as another tool in your weight loss tool belt. There is a lot of information that you can use to plan menus and select foods that you want to make part of your diet.

For more information on nutrition labels and the data they contain, check with your doctor or consult a nutritionist.

Monitoring Your Progress

Hopefully by now you have a fairly good idea of how you are going to go about losing your weight. Before we get into the actual CDO concept, we need to discuss one further element to a successful weight loss plan. That is monitoring your progress.

No one can expect to make a long journey without checking a road map from time to time. We all need to know if we are on the right track and that we are moving ahead according to schedule. If something goes wrong somewhere along the route, the faster we realize it, the easier it is to make a mid course correction.

Monitoring your progress is easy if you have taken the time to create some realistic goals. Once you have your goals you can compare your weight to where you should be and see if you are on schedule, ahead of schedule or behind schedule. Then, depending on where you are, you can make adjustments.

If you don't have goals, seriously consider developing some. It makes it so much easier and so much more accurate than just comparing weight to goal. There are so many factors that need to be considered and goals just make it so much easier.

One common question is "How often should I weigh myself?" This might be different so everyone because some of us get upset at every little change while others just don't care from one day to the next.

I am not so sure that frequency is as important as the time that you weight yourself. It is important to weight yourself the same time every day. Not to the minute of course but within a few hours.

The reason for this is that your weight will vary during the day. You will weigh less in the morning when you wake up than you did when you went to bed for example. So don't compare today's morning weight with tomorrow's evening weight. That is not an accurate comparison. Keep it the same time each day for the most accurate comparison.

While some people like to weight themselves 43 times a day, it really makes sense to just weigh yourself once a day or every other day. Keep a record of it and over a week or so you will get a pretty good indication of how things are going.

Weight will vary according to what you eat and what you do each day.

If you eat a lot of food high in sodium (salt) you will retain more water and your weight will go up for a day or so.

Then you will lose the water weight and your real weight will come through.

Naturally the more you eat in a day the more food weight you will have as well. To take that one step further, if you weigh yourself before you use the bathroom, for example, you might weigh more than after you used the bathroom. That's enough information there. You get my drift!

They key is to understand whether or not you are making progress. Do not judge based on a day or two of weight measurements. But if at the end of the week you are the same weight, or more, that you were at the end of the week before, we might have to change things.

The earlier we know if we are on track the easier it is to make adjustments. People who eat too much for a MONTH before weighing themselves will have a month of overeating to make up for. Someone who finds out in a day or two can easily make an adjustment quickly.

The data you get from your monitoring need not be shared with anyone. It is for your own use to tell you whether or not what you are doing is effective. Personally I think you should share it with your doctor so he or she can make sure you are doing things at the right pace. Losing weight too quickly can be dangerous for some people.

Whatever your goals might be, be sure to monitor your progress. It will keep you motivated, on track and will give you better results with less effort.

Goals & Mini-Goals

As with many things in life, a goal is something that we either aspire to achieve or that we are tasked with. An example of a goal we are tasked with might be to achieve a 50% growth in sales next year at work. An example of a goal we aspire to achieve might be to be able to run a marathon within 2 years or to complete college in the next two years.

In this book we are going to concentrate on the goals WE place in our lives not the ones given to us by others. When it comes to weight loss, goals are very important and actually help keep us focused and motivated. That is, when goal setting is done responsibly.

Goals are at their most effective when they are reasonable and achievable. If you set a goal so large and so impossible that you are bound to fail, you will not be motivated to achieve that goal. But when goals are realistic and achievable, they can be a powerful motivator.

Goals also give us a way to measure our progress. When we see ourselves making progress in anything, we get excited and re-motivated to keep up our efforts. In other words, goals let us see our progress and keep ourselves on track. Not only that, but they let us know whether what we are doing is working or if we have to make changes.

But in order to remain effective, goals must be reasonable, achievable, and the time frame has to be short enough for us to remain motivated. The goal also cannot appear to be so large that we become intimidated by it.

For example, if we need to lose 100 pounds, setting a goal to lose 100 pounds might appear to be so large we would immediately become overwhelmed and disenchanted. Plus, the gains we might make on a weekly basis would seem to be such a small part of the goal we might just quit. In other words, the entire task would be overwhelming to us.

A far better way to set our goals is to break up our goals into "bite sized" pieces that would appear more achievable and possible. In the case of our 100 pound weight loss example above, we would take that 100 pound goal and break it down into 10 – 10 pound "mini-goals. Each mini-goal would carry a shorter completion date.

Think about the ways this is so much better for us. First, if we lost 5 pounds towards our 100 pounds that is just 5% of our huge goal but 50% of our first mini-goal.

The progress we made is more clearly shown in the mini-goal. The more we see progress the motivated we are to keep doing what we are doing.

Second, in order to keep motivated, we should always celebrate our successes and achievements along the way. Mini goals allow us to celebrate more often and get us to feel good about what we are doing. The better we feel about what we are doing, the more motivated we become.

Third, and this is very important, mini goals allow us to more accurately measure our progress. Trying to gauge progress over a long period of time towards a single goal might be difficult. But when a large goal is broken down into smaller goals, we can see how long it took to complete each one. This will uncover some hidden problems or issues that might need to be addressed. The end result is that we will become more aware, more motivated and more engaged.

Mini goals are especially useful when it comes to weight loss. When you start a new weight loss program you lose more weight in the beginning than you will at the end. With one goal you will see rapid weight loss in the beginning but see that slowly go down over time. This might lead you to think you are doing something wrong when in fact it is just nature.

Mini goals help this because you can assign different time lines to each mini goal. For example, let's say you break your weight loss into 10 mini goals.

You can set your first mini goal at 5 pounds in two weeks. But your last 2 mini goals might be 1 pound in 2 weeks because it gets harder and harder to lose weight near the end. This will help keep you motivated.

Now I need to say something important right now. A lot of you might think this is all kind of BS and that a goal is a goal no matter how big. 100 pounds is the same as 10-10 pound goals. But remember that we are dealing with the human brain and our brains take a whole lot of things into consideration when it evaluates things.

Little things like emotions and perceptions and feelings that all come together to either create a positive or negative outlook on something. When it comes to weight loss, the beginning is tough but it gets easier when you see the benefits of what you are doing.

It might take a few weeks or months before you fit into that pair of pants or dress you want to wear but a mini goal will get you motivated and show your progress every week. Motivation is everything in the beginning. We want to work through that time where we are still thinking about what we are doing. We need to remain motivated until the things we are doing become habits.

If breaking up a goal sounds trivial and foolish, it is not. Anything that helps us to from where we are to where we want to be is not trivial. Instead, mini goals should be viewed as a very important weight loss tool that helps us achieve our goals. Foolish or not, they work and you should give them a try.

Goals are not Etched In Stone!

The last thing we need to discuss when it comes to our goals is that they are not etched in stone.

Our goals can and should be adjusted as we move forward. Sometimes we might set an overly ambitious goal and have to adjust it to make it achievable. Sometimes an injury or other unforeseen event makes it impossible to continue what we are doing for a while.

Whatever the reason, we should spend a few minutes every so often and go over our goals and make adjustments as needed. Now I am not saying we goof off and not do what we should and just adjust the goal so we can meet it. What I am saying is that you need to be honest with yourself and understand when something is too difficult or when something changes.

Maybe you get the flu and have to stop exercising. Maybe there is a vacation scheduled and that takes you away from the gym or puts you in an environment where you eat things you normally wouldn't.

Hey, we are all human and we all deserve a break and a little reward now and then. Just use our goals as a way to stay on track and monitor our progress. Our goals are tools we use to achieve objectives. Don't let them frustrate you or cause you to get depressed. Use them as motivators and adjust them as necessary.

When designed and used properly, goals can be a great way to getting to the finish line faster and with far less wasted effort.

Goals will help keep you on track and will also let you know when something is going the wrong way. Goals are all part of our knowledge of where we are and where we want to be. The more knowledge we have, the greater our chances of success.

So let's take some time to create a reasonable and achievable set of goals and then use them to help us along the way!

Creating New Behaviors

Before we move on, we have to take a moment to agree on something. The fact that you want to, or need to, lose weight now is because of things you have done in the past. You either gained weight because you ate too much, ate the wrong kinds of foods, or were not active enough.

This is not meant to assess blame or make you feel bad. Instead, it is designed to get you to accept responsibility for your current weight. You weigh what you weigh because you have done what you've done.

Now that we agree on that (hopefully!) we need to agree on one more thing. If your current behaviors got you into your current weight, then those same behaviors are not going to get you to your new weight. That just makes sense, doesn't it?

For example, if you earn $100 a week but spend $200, you will go into debt. You will stay in debt, even go deeper in debt, if you continue to spend more than you make. The same goes for weight loss. You cannot eat the same, get the same exercise, and expect those same behaviors to produce different results.

So we can now agree that in order to lose weight, and keep that weight off, we need to change some behaviors. Without changing the behaviors we cannot expect or get a different outcome. With that in mind, let's get started figuring out what needs to be done.

First of all, we should stress again the importance of being honest with yourself. We all have strong and weak points and we need to understand what those might be so we can address the weaker points and use those strong points.

For example, many of us overeat when we are stressed out or upset. If we have problems at work, or with a relationship, or if anything is not going right for us, a LOT of people find comfort in food. Unfortunately, comfort foods are usually not salads or healthy foods. Instead they are the high fat and high calorie foods like burgers, fries, ice cream, cookies and other similar foods.

I am sure you can look back at a time when you were experiencing something stressful and you sat down in front of the television and downed an entire bag of chips.

Or maybe drowned your sorrows in a 5 scoop ice cream sundae with all the toppings.

As we said, a LOT of people do this kind of thing and you should not be embarrassed about it. This is not about blame it is about realizing what we are doing and correcting it.

Ask yourself what you do that might influence how successful you are with your weight loss. Look at your food journal (remember that, right?) and see if any patterns exist. Do you eat more when you are angry, upset or stressed? When are you more likely to eat high calorie foods? Do you snack a lot before bedtime? Do you often hit fast food places for lunches or snacks? Knowing what you do is the first step. So do some thinking and write down what you think you do that is making you gain weight.

While it is easy to say "just stop it" when it comes to bad or negative habits, that just doesn't work. The reason is if we try to stop doing something, that requires willpower and constant focus and we all know by now that this just does not work.

But what if we recognize a bad behavior and substitute a good one? What if we make a conscious effort to go out for a walk when we feel stressed or angry? What if we bring something tasty with us for lunch instead of hitting the fast food places when we get those cravings? Those late night snacks? Maybe we make it a new habit to get some exercise at night which will also make us sleep better at the same time?

The key is to take our bad behaviors and substitute good ones in their place. Not all at once of course but over time.

If you are an emotional eater, becoming more aware of this and substituting something different will go a long way in getting you back on track and keeping you that way.

One thing is 100% certain, if you keep on doing the exact things that made you heavy in the first place, you will not be successful in your weight loss goals. You might achieve some short-term success but you will be far more likely to put all that weight back on and more.

Another way of looking at this might be to view the situations and emotions that make us eat as things that make us work harder to achieve our goals. By taking corrective action, we will be making our weight loss easier and less stressful. And we all know that easier and less stressful is a good thing.

So take a long and hard look at what you do under certain situations. Be honest with yourself and remember that no one need see what you write down or what your weaknesses might be. This is completely between you and yourself. No one else. So be honest and try and identify those areas that need change,

Then find something you enjoy, or that is better for yourself, and substitute that in place of the bad behavior. The more you do this the more you will regain control over your life.

Before closing this chapter, we also need to touch on one more subject. That is mental health.

Some of us may have emotional issues that cause us to over eat. Some of these issues may be quite severe and may not respond to our attempts to deal with them.

We might need help. Some of these issues can be very deep seated in our brains and require outside assistance. If this is the case, I urge you to seek help.

There is no shame or embarrassment in getting professional help. With proper help you can effectively deal with these situations and make your life better and stronger. This is not just about weight loss but about your entire life. If you feel you do need help, get it. Your doctor can advise you on whom to see for your specific problem.

Water –A Key Weight Loss Ingredient!

A critical part of ever healthy lifestyle is making sure the body gets all the water it needs before it needs it. Failure to properly hydrate the body can cause all kinds of problems from muscle cramps to kidney problems.

Many people think it is smart to reduce the amount of water because water means weight. They think it is great to lose 4 pounds during a run or walk because that is all sweat and now you weigh 4 pounds less.

Well, I've got news for you! You did not burn 14,000 calories (4 pounds X 3,500 calories) in that walk! You lost water weight due to sweating and exertion. You need to replace that water so your body and continue to provide the chemical actions that go on inside your body.

We also said in a paragraph about that we need to make sure we give our bodies the water they need BEFORE they need it.

That means drinking water before you workout and continuing to drink during your exercise and after wards as well. This will allow your body to function properly. I read one doctor say if you wait until you're thirsty, you waited too long!

Our muscles and systems need water to function properly. You cannot expect a dehydrated body to be able to continue to function let alone exercise. Left unaddressed, dehydration can cause passing out and even death!

It has long been said that the average person should drink 6-8 glasses of water every day. This is the figure for average people with average exercise levels. Someone who exercises or sweats a lot needs MORE that those 6-8 glasses each day. They might need 10-12 or more depending on what they do and where they do it.

Let's get one thing very clear right now, though.

When we refer to getting 6-8 glasses of water a day, we mean WATER! We do not count beer or soda or fruit juices or flavored drinks. Water is the very best drink for overall body health. It contains no calories, artificial sweeteners and none of the crap that is in those processed drinks we all drink.

And a word about soda and alcohol too. Alcohol actually dehydrates you as you drink! The more alcohol you drink the more water you need as well.

Soda is another drink that actually dehydrates you as you drink it. Soda has a lot of salt in it. It's designed to make you thirsty so you will drink more of it! For every can or either regular or diet soda you drink, you should ADD one glass of water to your daily requirement!

Benefits of Drinking Water

Drinking water has other benefits as well for our weight loss plan. First of all, water has no calories but it takes calories for the body to process it and run it through our digestive systems. So drinking water helps us burn calories and lose weight!

The other important thing water does is help flush toxins and by products from our bodies. This helps keep our bodies clean of these substances and helps it function at a higher level.

How to Get Enough Water

Some people have a hard time getting their 6-8 glasses of water a day. Not because it is difficult but because they just don't think about it or count what they drink.

For those people, the best thing to do is to keep a jug of cold water in the refrigerator and drink from it throughout the day.

You might even be right that drinking cold water requires more calories to process but the main reason is that the jug lets you know how close or how far you are away from your 6-8 glasses. If the jug isn't empty, you are not finished yet!

You can substitute water for soda or wine at meals as well. This has a double effect because you should be adding to your 6-8 glasses for the soda and alcohol that you drink throughout the day! So changing to water will help you make your 6-8 glasses go easier and faster.

If you have questions about how much water you should drink every day, be sure to check with your doctor. He or she will be able to give you more information and guidance.

What Exactly is Calorie Deficit Optimization?

Calorie Deficit Optimization is what we call combining diet, exercise and behavior modification in such a way that we accomplish the weight loss process with less stress, effort and sacrifice.

We found that diet and exercise alone do not give you the best chances for success. Plus, diet and exercise are sometimes not that easy or enjoyable for some people. Because of this we sought to design a system where everything we do is geared towards one common goal. That goal is to make the weight loss process easier, more enjoyable and longer lasting.

The CDO weight loss plan is a plan designed so that everybody can be successful and lose the weight they want to lose. Even more important, if you follow the plan the weight you lose will come off and stay off.

That is a huge upgrade over conventional diets where you lose weight and then put all the weight back on later. When you follow the CDO plan, the weight comes off and stays off!

The plan also realizes that the easier we make something, there will be more people being successful and more people sticking with it no matter how long it might take. We also realize that if something is made easier, more people will try it.

This is not some pie in the sky gimmick or voodoo or any of that nonsense. Instead it is a program designed to achieve success not through massive change and sacrifice but rather through adding the benefits of small changes to produce big results.

The CDO program is flexible as well. We find that the more options and control you give someone, the more they will apply themselves and the greater their success will be. Everyone is different and what might work for me might not work that well for you. So we allow you to choose the things you do and how your do them. You are in control and you make the choices!

We all know that if you want to lose weight you need to burn more calories than you take in. That is just basic science. But there are so ways to accomplish this that you will almost definitely find the best way for you personally.

The CDO plan is easy as well. We show you how to accomplish more in a healthy and safe manner without sweat pouring exercise or starvation diets.

We show you how to design a plan that will not only help you lose the weight but always take steps to keep that weight from coming back.

This book is divided into two sections. The first part of the book lays the framework for developing your plan and explains all the little yet important things you can do to increase weight loss while minimizing effort. Every chapter is important and we hope you will read and follow every one. Even if something sounds silly or even stupid, we would like you to know that it serves a valid purpose. So please don't skip over any of these preparation chapters.

The second part of the book is the CDO plan itself and the explanation of its parts. Here you will learn how to use everything you learned in part one to create a powerhouse program that is both easy to follow yet effective. We will show you how to get better results with less effort.

Before we get started, let me say again we are not doctors. We are not medical experts and make no claims regarding medical issues in this program. We trust that you will make this program part of your health improvement plan and that you will consult your doctor before starting any kind of exercise or weight loss column.

There are so many medical issues, diseases and factors involved that we could never cover all in one book. So please consult your family doctor before starting CDO or any other plan. Show your doctor this book and get their opinion on it first.

OK! Let's get started.....................

CDO: Getting Started

This is where it all comes together. This is where we finally get started on our journey to get to the weight we really want. This part is critical to your success so PLEASE do not skip over parts of this because you think they don't matter. Trust me, they do!

Step 1: Understand WHY You Want to Do This!

Really understand why you are doing this in the first place. Be honest with yourself. Take time to write down all the benefits you will receive if you complete your goals.

What will you be able to do after you lose weight that you can't now? How different will you look? How much better will you feel? What do you expect to get out of this entire process? Write it down as descriptively as possible.

Be as specific as you can. For example, instead of "get in better shape" write down "be able to run a 5K race" or "be able to walk 5 miles" or "be able to play 3 sets of tennis". Another example might be "want clothes to fit better" might be written down as "fit into the brown pants that I haven't been able to wear in 3 years."

Visualize as much as possible. See yourself running that race or walking that walk or playing that third set of tennis. See yourself thinner and easily sliding into those pants. Make it as real as possible. Visualization is something we will use throughout the program to keep you motivated.

Step 2: Decide Your Weight Goals

You can't start a journey if you don't know where you are going. The same applies to weight loss. The plan to lose 5 pounds will be much different than the plan to lose 100 pounds. Think about how much weight you want to lose. Discuss this with your doctor to make sure this is a safe and healthy goal. After all, a person can be too skinny.

Make sure this goal is realistic. Remember goals are adjustable and if things go better or worse they can be changed. You always want an achievable goal in front of you so that you will continue to believe you can accomplish it. If the goal is so "out there" that you know you won't achieve it, you will be more likely to give up.

Step 3: Decide on a Time Frame

While weight loss should never be rushed or considered a race to the finish, sometimes there are time concerns involved. For example, if your motivation is to fit into a special dress for your sister's wedding, you need to reach your goal by the time of the wedding. If you reach your goal 2 years after the wedding that's great but it will not help you when the wedding comes around!

Time frames also need to be reasonable and healthy. Too rapid a weight loss can cause medical problems and health issues. Again, when you talk to your doctor, discuss your weight loss goals and time frames with them. They will let you know what is safe for you. Always remember that the guidelines in this book are only suggestions for the sake of examples and may or may not be right for you.

Also, make the time frame achievable as well. You need to honestly believe you can achieve the goals in the time allotted or you will not stay motivated. For example, if you have to lose 100 pounds and you say you will do that in a month, that's just ridiculous! It might take you 2 years to lose that weight. Unless there is something compelling or critical about a specific time frame, do it smart and healthy and take your time.

Speaking of time, here is another thing to carefully consider. If you have a specific goal or deadline for losing your weight, do not wait too long to get started.

Weight loss almost always takes a little longer than you think and you want to give yourself plenty of time. So if that special wedding is a year away and you need to lose 25 pounds, don't wait 10 months to start! Start now! Remember that weight loss is beneficial in a lot of ways and losing the weight early is a good thing anyway!

To lose weight in a healthy and responsible fashion, you should not try to lose more than 1-2 pounds a week. The first few weeks you might lose more because of water weight and other factors but once things "stabilize" a 1-2 pound weekly weight loss is the most you should aim for. Again, check with your doctor to find out what is the best weight loss rate for your situation. Remember, they know best.

Step 4: Know What Your Weight Gain Is Per Week or Month

It is important to understand how much weight you have gained over the last month or year. Knowing how much weight you gain in a certain time frame can help you understand how much you have to reduce your diet or increase your exercise to make that weight loss reverse itself.

For example, if you gain an average of one pound per week, that means you either have to reduce your calorie intake by 3,500 or increase your exercise by 3,500 just to stop the weight gain. If you gained 2 pounds a week, you have to make up 7,000 calories.

We need to know this so we can figure out how to meet both our weight loss and time frame goals without making things are harder than we need to. If your weight gain or loss was different over a month or two, try and remember what you weighed last year and use that figure. The longer period of time we use the more accurate the number should be.

Step 5: Go Over Your Food Journal

Hopefully you created your food journal like we advised. This is very important because it helps provide you with some ideas on how best to achieve your goals with a minimum of sacrifice or hardship. Remember, we are looking for the easiest yet most responsible way to lose the weight we need to lose. So if you have not created your food journal yet, please stop and do so now. It will become more important as we go on.

Look in your journal for the highest calorie foods you eat or the times when you binge eat. See if there is something you can substitute for these high calorie foods. If these are meals, substitute a turkey sandwich or a piece of chicken for that burger and fries. If it's a snack, substitute some carrot sticks for the potato chips. Even changing that ice cream you love for a frozen yogurt or low fat ice cream can help.

Write down the number of calories you think you can reduce in your diet without undergoing a huge sacrifice.

Again, be realistic. Do NOT underestimate the size portions you eat and do not over estimate the number of calories you think you are cutting out by changing or eliminating something. This is YOUR plan to reach YOUR goals. Fooling yourself will hurt no one but you. Be as accurate an honest as possible with every judgment and decision you make.

Step 6: Determine Your Current Exercise Level

Now we want an honest assessment of the amount of exercise you get in an average day. If you took our advice and purchased or used a pedometer to measure how much you walk in a given day, that's great because it gives you a pretty good idea of where you are right now.

Include exercise at the gym, any walking or running or sports you get involved in or any work normally done around the house. Cleaning the house or mowing the lawn burns calories! You could take 5,000 steps to mow the lawn! Even cooking a meal is said to burn 110 calories an hour.

We need to understand our current exercise level so we know how much we need to increase the amount of exercise to reach our goals. This is important because some people work out every day for two hours and still gain weight because they eat a ton of calories. It would not be reasonable to expect these people to increase exercise.

Yet other people lead almost exercise free lives and although they ear relatively little in the way of calories, they burn off fewer and they gain weight. You need to understand where you fall between those two extremes.

There are charts available online for the number of calories burned in an hour for just about any exercise. So if you play tennis for two hours, count those calories because even though tennis is enjoyable, it still counts as exercise!

Again, BE HONEST when it comes to these assessments. Do not give yourself credit for more exercise than you get. This will only reduce your progress and increase the time it takes you to reach your goals, it can also get you frustrated when you don't see the expected progress.

Step 7: Let's Figure Out Where We Stand Right Now

Now we have all the pieces of the puzzle we need to use to determine what we need to do in order to stop weight gain and then get ourselves to lose weight. We are going to take the amount of weight we gain each week and convert that into calories (# of pounds X 3,500). This will give us the number of calories we have to reduce or burn off to get us to **stop** gaining weight.

Then we are going to take our weight loss weekly goal (the 1-2 pounds) and convert that into calories. (1-2 pounds X 3,500 = 3,500 -7,000 calories). We are going to add the calories from the first step to this number of calories:

One-half pound a week average weight gain - 1,750 calories

One pound weight loss each week- 3,500 calories

Total calories needed to reduce- 5,250 calories

So now we know we are going to have to reduce our weekly diet or increase our weekly exercise by 1,750 calories to stop losing weight and by 5,250 calories to lose one pound a week.

This gives you a solid idea of what needs to be done to get from where you are to where you want to be. You know with a fairly accurate number what you need to do to achieve success. Knowledge is power and knowledge helps us make decisions that are good and practical.

The entire information gathering process should have taken you about 15 minutes if you had followed the suggestions up to this point. If you did not create a food journal, or if you did not track your exercise, then you have to do that for at least one week (2 or more is better and more accurate) in order to get the required information.

Having this information will enable you to create an initial plan to get you back on track without excessive sacrifice and effort. No one likes sacrifice and no want wants to keep on sacrificing. So if we can minimize, possible even eliminate sacrifice with a reasonable and information-based program, won't you agree that is a good thing to do?

So now we have our number of calories in hand. So what do we do with it? That's next!

CDO Part One:

Synergy

For those of you who might not be familiar with the term synergy, it refers to multiple things having a greater impact when used together than they would have if they had been used separately. Sort of like 2+2=5!

With CDO we take several little things and combine them to produce hugely effective results with much less effort. While that sounds like a line of crap, let me assure you that this does work. For now you will have to trust us but once you give CDO a chance, you will become convinced!

By combining several things into our weight loss plan, we can create a plan that works well without subjecting us to a lot of unnecessary stress, sacrifice and effort. Remember willpower is a myth when it comes to long term results. We want to find a way to accomplish a goal that requires less effort.

We want to figure out a way to lose our weight without a lot of pain and sacrifice.

We do that by combining things like diet, exercise, motivation, knowledge, substitution, behavior modification and creating something that is effective, produces great results and most of all, just plain works. Though each of these individual items are important, when you combine them they produce far greater results than they would if used individually. That's what makes this program work so well for most people.

We take all of these individual factors and use them together to reduce effort, to reduce stress, to reduce sacrifice and to actually help us help ourselves in reaching our goals. If it sounds too good to be true, it really isn't.

With all of this in mind, and with all of us excited and ready to get started, let's get started with The CDO Weight Loss Plan!

CDO Part Two:

What Do You Want to Do?

The greatest part of the CDO weight loss plan is that it puts YOU in total control. This is not a rigid and fixed type program but rather a program that can grow and change with you so it continues to fit your needs even when goals and situations change. In other words, it is a customer designed adaptable weight loss plan with you as the captain.

So now is the time where YOU get to decide HOW you want to proceed. There are a few decisions to make but they are easy and any of them can be changed at any time. Again, there is no time limit on your weight loss unless YOU want there to be. Se we concentrate on results not arbitrary deadline.

Step One: Understand What Needs to Happen

Understand how many calories you have to either burn or reduce through diet to get you to stop gaining weight and also the number you need to start losing weight.

These two numbers are important because they relate to how much you have to do to hit your goals. Knowing the number of calories in will take to stop gaining weight is important because you can use that number for those tough weeks when you are on vacation or during the holidays or special occasions.

But the number that we need to lose weight is the number of calories we have to plan for. That is the number that will bring you to your goals or at least get you started in the right direction.

Step Two: Which Approach Is Best for You???

To get rid of those "extra" calories, we have a choice. We can eat less or we can burn more calories. Some of us find the process of dieting extremely difficult and unappealing so we might want to go the exercise route. Others might find exercise unappealing and decide to do everything through diet.

The smart people, however, decide to accomplish their weight loss through a combination of diet and exercise. But the ultimate decision is up to you. This is your program and you are the captain!

Adding more exercise though has some great benefits. It raises our metabolism which causes us to burn more calories throughout the day even when we are not exercising. That can add up to a serious number of "bonus" calories at the end of the week! That makes you have to work less and working less always helps you stick to things longer and increases your odds of success!

Exercise also burns stored energy in the fat within our bodies. So even if you find yourself not losing the weight as fast as you want, it could be because you are turning fat into muscle. Muscle weighs more than fat so a better indication of progress might be how your clothes fit or how you look.

A great deal depends on the number of calories that you have to either reduce or burn away. If it is 500 calories, maybe diet will work. But if it is 7,000 calories, a combination of diet and exercise is the only really realistic choice.

This does not mean that you cannot achieve your goal by diet or exercise alone. What it does mean is that it will be EASIER if you do both. If, for some reason you cannot diet, or you cannot exercise, we can work through that. But if both are possible, then it will be easier for you if you choose both diet and exercise as your approach.

Step 3: Identify Dietary Opportunities

If you have not done so already, go through your food journal and identify potential savings and opportunities.

At this point we don't have to act on all of them, just list them so you know what you will have to work with.

For example, if you come up with 10 things you can do that will save you 200 calories a week each, that represents a potential savings of 2,000 calories every week.   Try and be honest and realistic and come up with real calorie savings not inflated figures to make things look better than they really are!

Step 4: Identify Exercise Options

Next is trying to identify what types of exercise are available to you. We talked a lot about walking and this is a great way to get exercise. You can do it anywhere and there is no cost to start, either.

But we have sports like tennis and handball, bowling, running, baseball or softball or any physical activity. Once you have a list of these activities, do an online search to find the average number of calories you will burn for each hour you do that activity.

Take each activity and figure out a reasonable amount of time that you intend to do that activity every week. Be specific and be accurate. Tend to measure on the very conservative side. For example, if you think you might walk 4 hours a week, consider counting it as 3 hours. This will allow you to miss a day when something comes up. If you do the 4 hours you will just lose more weight and that's not a bad thing anyway.

Step 5: How Will You Do It?

Now you need to decide how you are going to achieve your goal. If you have decided on a combination of diet and exercise, how are you going about splitting things up? If you can easily identify a few dietary changes that can save you 2,000 calories a week out of, say, a 3,500 calorie need then you would have to burn off the remaining 1,500 calories.

Decide which you think is best for you and then determine how you will handle the number of calories you need to lose weight. Eat more or exercise more, it's up to you.

Sometimes, especially if you have to make some serious changes, it might be best to gradually go into things a little bit. Take a couple of weeks to get used to things and gradually add more into the mix. Time is not as important as your overall success.

Now that you know the average number of calories you need to address, add your dietary changes and exercise expectations. If they add up to more than the number of calories you needed, you're in great shape! You might be able to cut back some on the diet and/or exercise if that is the case. If the calories do not add up, you either have to cut back on some more foods or get more exercise to get to where you need.

At this point we are trying to make an educated guess as to what we have to do to reach our goals.

This is not a guessing game. We have spent some real time and effort figuring out what we need to do. How accurate we are has yet to be determined but we have a reasonable starting point.

So here we are. We have gathered the information we need and made some tough decisions based on what we want and what we like. We have developed a plan that should meet our needs with a minimum of stress and effort. So we are ready for the last phase.

CDO Part Three:

Monitoring & Recalibration

We have come such a long way since we first decided to lose weight and the fact that you have come so far speaks greatly of your dedication and motivation. Making changes is not easy and we have done our best to make it as easy as possible with a minimum amount of sacrifice. But it still takes a little bit of work especially at the beginning.

At this point the key to our success is in our ability to monitor our progress and "recalibrate" or adjust our plans as needed. This is important because so far we have done things largely on an intellectual level. What I mean by that is that what we have done so far looks great on paper and should work very well.

But the human body and the human mind can do some things that we are not prepared for and even a few things that come totally unexpected. Now most of the time these little setbacks or added factors can be dealt with easily. But this can be done easily only if we remain vigilant and keep on the lookout for them. If we don't do that, they can go on for weeks, even months, without us knowing about them. This sets our progress way back and can even lead to complete failure and loss of motivation.

Even if nothing out of the ordinary or unexpected happens, your body will also change over time and those changes will affect your weight loss. As you body loses fat and water weight, your weight loss will slow down. This does not mean you are doing anything wrong, it is just how the body reacts. So when these things happen, we often need to re-evaluate our plans and make some mid course corrections.

Here are a few things you really need to do to enable you to catch problems or outside factors early:

Follow Your Plan

We spent a lot of time learning about ourselves and the weight loss process. We spent more time gathering information and learning about why we want to lose the weight and how to best go about it. All this leads to the creation of a weight loss plan that fits our personality and desires and our long-term goals.

But our plan will only be as good as the person following it. If we follow the plan and do not cheat or slack off, we should lose the weight we want to in a very easy and stress free manner. But if we leave the plan in a drawer someplace and just go it alone, our results will be less, the effort and sacrifice greater and you will have a far greater chance of just plain giving up.

So make it a priority to follow your plan closely. Especially in the beginning when everything is new to you. Your plan is like a guide or roadmap and you will be able to refer back to it until much of it is imprinted in your memory. Even after you have it all down in your mind, you plan will provide you with mini-goals that will help you monitor your progress and keep you on track.

Weigh Yourself Often

I'm not one of those people who weight themselves 87 times a day. That really doesn't tell you much and it can frustrate you because of fluctuations in your weight throughout the day.

So when we say "often" we do not mean every 20 minutes. Once a day is plenty. Try to weight yourself the same time every day because body weight does change during the day. You will likely weigh a little more at night than you do in the morning.

You will weigh more after a meal than you weighed before you ate. Some people weigh themselves every other day or maybe just twice a week.

Whatever frequency you choose, make sure you weigh yourself the same time each time.

All of this is normal and all you really need to concentrate on is weighing yourself the same time each day so you are comparing legitimate and accurate weights. Naturally the easiest times are when you wake up and when you go to bed. Again, pick one or the other. But do not compare your night time weight yesterday with your morning weight tomorrow. The result will be distorted.

If possible, keep a chart of your weight. This might come in handy spotting trends when you lost more or less than what you thought you would lose. Again, information is knowledge and being able to see more of what you are doing and the results you receive can be helpful.

Monitor Your Results & Health Weekly

Along with your weight loss (or gain) every week, you should also monitor your overall health and how you feel as well. These factors can help you adjust your plan, your workouts and your goals to get optimum results.

A lot of people keep a journal and this can prove very helpful. In your journal write down the "hard facts" such as weight loss, exercise types and times and other aspects of your plan.

Write down any holidays or special events that might have caused you to go off your diet. This is done not to make you feel bad or to assess blame but only to explain a difference in weight loss. Sometimes we tend to forget these things so writing them down is important.

Also write down how you felt during the week. Were you tired all the time? Did you have any aches or pains or physical issues? How well did you sleep? All of these things matter because they could be signs of exercising too much or too hard. They could also signal not eating enough calories for your body to safely function.

If you have a blood pressure monitor, keep a log of your blood pressure. You will probably notice it going down as you lose and start exercising. This is your body telling you that things are working and it is now operating more efficiently.

If you are a diabetic, make sure you check your blood glucose levels often. Exercise will tend to change the way your body metabolizes glucose and you should see your glucose levels fall as you lose weight and exercise. This could cause you to require less medication so be sure to make your doctor aware of any low sugar reactions that might occur. I experienced a lot of them when I started because the body was just working better. A reduction in meds and everything was great!

Always keep in mind that you are not only losing weight but getting your body to function better and to feel better at the same time. If this is not working, or if you feel bad, or if you hurt, or if your body is sending you a message that something is wrong, do NOT ignore it!

Make Corrections When Necessary

The body is a complicated structure. A LOT of things go on inside and sometimes the results we get are not what we expected. Sometimes this is good and sometimes this is bad. We need to accept these situations and learn how to deal with them.

Our plan might tell us we need to do certain things and the results should be 2 pounds of weight loss per week. The reality might be that we lose 4 pounds! Or, in some cases, we might not lose any weight at all! If this happens one week, make note of it but do not panic or get frustrated. Watch things for another week and see if things so back to normal. If your weight loss returns to the desired levels, you don't have to do anything.

But if you are losing weight too rapidly, or not at all, you need to change your diet and exercise levels to get things moving. If you are losing weight too rapidly, add some calories to your diet. I prefer to leave exercise at the current level because exercise has so many benefits outside of weight loss. As long as you are not hurting or over tired, leave exercise alone!

Try and make minor changes with diet to see if that can bring you back to where you need to be. If you feel you are not doing as much exercise as you should, by all means increase it but try to limit such increases to no more than a 10% increase per week. We do not want to overburden or injure our muscles and joints.

It is just important at this point to make sure we know what is going on and become aware of any questionable things that are going on. This way we can make corrections or address issues quickly and limit their consequences.

Adjust Goals When Required

Sometimes you goals are just too ambitious or something changes to make them unrealistic. One of the most common things that many people experience is a slowdown in weight loss as we get further into our diet and exercise program.

This happens for several reasons. One of the reasons is that as we become lighter, it takes less calories to move us through our daily routine. At the same time, our bodies are getting more in shape and more efficient so it takes fewer calories for us to accomplish certain tasks. It's cruel but true!

Another factor that almost everyone experiences is that it is just more difficult to lose pounds as we get further into our weight loss. That is because in the beginning we are losing loose fat and water weight.

But as we move forward, the body has to draw on its fat reserves and that fat has been there for years and years. Your body will also tend to fight this process as well thinking it is being starved. That is the reason why starvation diets and missing meals do not help weight loss.

Other things that make it difficult to achieve goals are honest misjudgments in what we are able or willing to do. We may really believe that we are capable of performing a certain amount of exercise each week but the body and spirit just are not willing.

Or, we are have overestimated calorie savings of eliminating certain foods. In any case, when results do not come sometimes goals need to be adjusted.

One very important thing to remember is that having to adjust a goal does not mean you have failed. What it means is that you realize the goal is no longer realistic and needs to be adjusted or reset. This happens in life all the time and successful people realize this and make adjustments.

Now you can just be lazy and not do the things you committed to and still change your goals. But if you do that, remember that you are cheating just one person. You.

You are the one who wants to lose the weight and you will be the one who will either be successful or not. So be honest. If you are not doing the things you should be doing, start doing them. Do not just adjust the goal to cover laziness.

But if you are doing the things you should, or if you find the going just too hard, please do not feel hesitant about adjusting your goals. Realistic goals help keep you motivated and engaged. Difficult goals threaten your commitment and your ability to stay motivated.

Remember the entire focus of this whole weight loss process has been on one thing. To get results in a manner that you can control and live comfortably with. Goals play an important part of this process. If you use goals correctly, you will get better results in a faster time frame. Keep them achievable, keep them realistic, and be honest with yourself and you will be successful.

Listen to Your Body!

Our bodies are remarkable works of art. They have complex systems that give us life and also provide the ability to think, be creative and make complex decisions. They also have the ability to communicate with us if we are receptive to listening.

When things are not going right, or when we do something our bodies have trouble with, our body lets us know. It might be pain or discomfort or it might be something that makes it difficult to continue like light headedness or even passing out. These are all reflexive actions our bodies take to protect itself. We just need to listen to our bodies more.

If we exercise and feel pain, we should cut back or stop. Pain is a way of telling us could be doing something wrong or that we have hurt something. Rapid heartbeat or extremely high blood pressure are other signs. Anytime we do not feel "right" we need to stop and listen to our bodies.

If you do feel bad, or just "not right", make sure you stop and see if the feeling passes. Sometimes we try to do too much too soon and our bodies cannot handle the stress or the effort. When we feel bad we need to stop and rest.

Constant hunger is not a good thing either. Hunger does not mean you are losing weight!

Hunger means your stomach is empty and your body wants or needs nourishment. Pay attention to these feeling and warning signs. Stay away from starvation diets and develop a plan that is healthy and gives the body plenty of good and healthy foods.

Most important, listen to your body when it says it needs water. Thirst is our body's way of telling us it is getting dehydrated. When you are thirsty you need to drink some water! Not soda, not beer, not wine but water. Water is essential to sustain life. So give your body the water it needs before it asks for it! Especially when you are exercising and sweating. Drink water before, during and after exercising so you don't get dehydrated.

Never ignore a body's message to you. Every feeling and ache and pain means something. Just listen and make sure you do everything in a healthy manner.

Take a Trip to the Bank!

Let's get ready to take flexibility to a whole new level! I mean whenever we can make something easier we grab at the chance, right? Well here's your chance to add a whole lot of flexibility to your CDO Weight Loss program!

We all have days when we feel better than others and also days where we are just "psyched" or in the mood to do things. On the flip side, we also have days when we don't want to do a damned thing and have little or no patience for anything. Well here is now we can take this and turn it into an advantage!

Get yourself a notebook, or make a page in your food journal book and create a "bank" page. On that page you will enter your weekly exercise goals and even your calorie goals. Then as each days goes by, if you should do MORE than your plan says you need to, you can write that down as a "deposit" in your exercise or food account.

For example, let's say your plan says you have to exercise enough to burn off 3,500 calories a week. That comes down to 500 calories a day. On Monday you exercise and burn off approx. 500 calories and that is good. But you feel really good on Tuesday and it is a gorgeous day so you walk a lot more or you play some more tennis and burn off 1,000 calories. Then you can take those 500 calories and make your "deposit" into your account.

That means you are 500 calories, or one day worth of exercise, ahead. So if you have an all day meeting or social event on Friday and will not be able to exercise, you already have those 500 calories in your account that you can "withdraw" on Friday!

This might sound a little silly or foolish but stop and think for a moment what this bank plan allows you to do.

It allows you to compensate for times when you cannot exercise

It allows for you to make calories for when you were sick.

It gives you more flexibility in your schedule
You can "bank" exercise calories to cover you through vacations.

If you exercise outside, it helps compensate for the weather.

It allows you to also make up for lost exercise.
It can function as a safety net for when you skip days

The end result is that you regain control in almost any situation. You now have more control over the present and the future. If it is more convenient to do more one day because another day is too packed to allow time for exercise, you don't have to lose that exercise; you have the ability to add that exercise into other days of that week.

The "bank" is just a fancy way to refer to a list of exercise and a running tally. But it gives you a way to make up for past times when you didn't do what you should have. Now you don't have to accept the lazy times but tell yourself instead that you now have to work harder to get back on track.

The bank is a way of keeping accountability without getting people so frustrated and depressed because they skipped a day (or a week). It also allows you to "bank" exercise in advance so you do not have to exercise while on vacation. Or at least not as much as you are supposed to.

There are two things you should be aware of when using the banking system.

The first is that it is never a good idea to overdo exercise. If you are used to walking one hour a day, you should not walk 10 hours the next day so you won't have to walk on vacation. Always keep your "extra" exercise within the healthy and safe range to avoid straining or hurting yourself.

The second thins has to do with your metabolism. Remember that exercise helps burn calories after you stop exercising. So you will get those extra minutes of calorie burning on days that you exercise. You will NOT get that on the days that you bank and skip.

So the bottom line is that exercise should be done on schedule whenever possible to get the most benefit and to remain in a healthy program. But we do acknowledge that sometimes we just cannot exercise for many reasons and this gives us a way to stay, or get back, on track without the guilt.

Food Bank

You can to the same thing with food calories but you need to be realistic and honest. If you know you have a wedding or big dinner coming up you can SLIGHTLY reduce your daily calorie intake to help bank calories so you wind up at goal at the end of the week.

Maybe that might mean skipping a mid day or nighttime snack and banking those 100 calories. The one thing you do NOT want to do is starve yourself for days to bank a large number of calories. That is not healthy and can be dangerous.

Do NOT skip meals and do NOT decrease the amount of calories consumed to extremely low levels. This is very important. Diets already lowered in calories should not be cut drastically more without medical supervision and approval!

Basically we want to give you the flexibility to save a few calories here and there to compensate for the occasional indulging. This can either be before the event if we know it is coming or after the event if it was unexpected.

Use, Not Abuse!

The purpose of the bank strategy is to give us a way to be flexible with our eating and exercise. It provides a way for us to accommodate special events, dinners out, and other situations while still staying on track at the end of the week or month. It provides us with a way of compensating for times of weakness and sickness as well.

But you should not be using this program as a way to increase your intake of high calorie meals and skipping of exercise. Your plan was designed to meet specific goals and it was created to do so in a healthy and responsible manner. So you not throw that plan out the window and make extensive use of the bank to do what you want when you want. That is not flexibility. That is not following your plan.

If you find yourself routinely banking large numbers of exercise or calories, it might be time to sit down and reassess your plan. Maybe you are in better shape and can do more exercise. Perhaps it is time to rebalance the calorie intake / exercise portion of the program.

Lastly, we must always remember that a critical part of the CDO plan is behavior modification. That means doing the things we need to do until they become part of our lifestyle and we do them automatically.

If we are constantly breaking the plan to eat fast food or high calorie meals and then starving ourselves to make up for it, that is NOT modifying our behavior. We will learn nothing from this way of doing things. For this, or any other, weight loss plan to work, we need to address and resolve the actions that made us overweight in the first place. That is where behavior modification comes in.

The banking program will provide you with more flexibility and a way to recover from special situations and vacations. It is a powerful tool to help fit things into your schedule while staying on track. It can eliminate excuses as well and that is an important factor too. Use the banking program as it is intended and you will find that it makes things a lot easier for you.

But if you use it too much, you will damage your chances of long term success.

Fads & Shortcuts

Weight loss is something that is very personal and very important to a lot of people. Because of this, there is a great market for anything that makes weight loss easier and faster. While there is nothing wrong with easier and faster, the problems occur when you start doing things that are unsafe or unhealthy.

We ask you that you step back whenever you see a product or a special diet that promises huge results and focuses on hype and promotion rather than sound medically sound weight loss. Some people and companies have just one goal in mind. That is to help you lose weight by removing some of your money from your wallet. I'm not saying their products will not work, only that you need to be skeptical and make sure they are healthy and safe to use.

I know I risk repeating myself again but when it comes to these "quick weight loss" products, it is crucial that you check with your doctor before going on any radical diet or ingesting any "magic" weight loss powder or drink.

There are a myriad of weight loss diets and products out there. From powders you pour in your bath water that claim to burn fat while you soak to a plastic suit that you wear when you sleep that causes you to lose weight. Now, do either of these products really work? If they do, are they healthy?

Wearing a plastic suit might help you wake up lighter but it's not because it burns off fat, it just makes you sweat more and you lose water weight. Water weight comes back as you hydrate yourself by drinking water throughout the day. I'm not sure how that bath powder works but anything that claims to make changes within your body needs to be absorbed into your body and that doesn't sound like something I want floating around inside me!

You will also see a lot of "fad" diets out there. The "celery diet", the "salad diet" and so on. All of these diets need to be scrutinized carefully to make sure they create a healthy and balanced diet. If you are expected to eat just one thing for breakfast lunch and dinner, you might lose weight but you could be missing important vitamins and minerals and nourishment.

Plus, these fad diets sometimes are just not sustainable. I mean how long can you eat salad three meals a day?

Personally, I would tire of that in a few days and would have nightmares about lettuce shortly afterwards! Calories are just one part of the weight loss equation. In order to lose weight, and keep it off, there are several other things you need to address. Fad diets usually don't touch on those things.

You may even think this CDO Weight Loss Plan is a fad. We can assure you that it is not. If you notice, nowhere in this book do we tell you specifically what to eat. Instead, we tell you to monitor what you eat and then make some minor corrections so your lose weight. We don't want or expect you to replace all your favorite foods with lettuce or tofu. We just want you to succeed.

We also address long-term weight loss and the need to change behaviors so you don't gain all that weight right back on when you stop. Fad diets don't address that. After you are sick of lettuce and start eating the triple cheeseburgers and large fries for lunch and dinner the pounds come right back.

There are also hundreds of machines and exercise systems out there designed to give you ripped abs and a tiny waist in only minutes per day. These are scientifically designed to work multiple muscle groups at the same time to produce quick results.

Well, let me give you one very important fact. Muscles only grow stronger through exercise
. Waists only get smaller through diet. These machines might give you the ability to do specific exercises but they require strenuous exercise in order to product those benefits. There are no "magic" machines out there that will produce a ripped and lean body without a heck of a lot of work.

Lastly, let me be very clear about something. Losing weight at too rapid a pace can be physically dangerous. Starvation diets can lead to bone and skeletal problems and other diseases and conditions as well. If you try to reduce your calorie intake too much, your body will not get what it needs when it needs it. Blood chemistry gets all out of whack and you energy level plummets. If you insist on using a plan that promises huge weight loss within a short time, PLEASE run it by your doctor first. It could be a life saving decision and a great use of your time.

The same goes for exercise. Rapid weight loss requires large reduction of calories PLUS large amounts of exercise. If you are very overweight, chances are you are not very active and not in great physical condition. We do not say this to offend you or make you feel bad. Instead, we are saying this to make you aware that you need to gradually introduce exercise into your daily life.

If you are used to sitting behind a desk all day and then go out and try to run 10 miles, you will not be able to do it and you can do some real damage to your heart and your body.

The same goes for doing 50 sit ups or for lifting heavy weights. All of these things can be dangerous for you if you do not do them gradually.

Fad diets and exercise gimmicks and weight loss powders and such are designed to get you to spend your money. The fact is, you don't have to spend a dime to lose weight safely.

In fact, if you want to lose weight safely and for the best long term results, here is all you need:

A pair of sneakers which you already own
A calorie counter book (less than $10)
A pedometer ($10-20)

A journal ($1)
One or Two Doctor Co-Pays ($25-$50)

Even the pedometer is optional but it is a great way to track you daily exercise. But the fact is, it should not cost you a lot of money to lose weight. In fact, the process will probably come out cheaper for you because you will spend less on food.

You don't need gimmicks and you don't need fad diets. Stay away from quick and easy and instead move over to smart and safe. Smart and safe will enable you to come out on top every single time.

Making CDO Work for You

We do things at our best in life when we are in control and we have a "say" in how things are done. No one likes to be dictated to. Few people like to be told there is none way, and just one way, to accomplish a goal. That is why most people fail. The CDO Weight Loss plan was developed to be a weight loss process where YOU have the most control. Because when YOU have control, YOU will do better and get better results.

That being said, there are some things YOU can do to make this entire journey more pleasurable and also help you get better results. Here are a few suggestions we have to make sure you are successful

Take Your Time!

I know this is the 42nd time I have said this but please take your time with your weight loss.

Do not rush it and do not do more than you should. Unless there are specific medical reasons why you need to accelerate the process, take it slow. Attaining your goal should be the primary focus of any weight loss program not how long it should take.

Slow and steady progress helps keep you motivated and engaged. Trying to do too much too fast is one of the most common reasons people fail at losing weight. Answer this question: What is better, losing 30 pounds in 12 months and being successful or trying to lose 30 pounds in 3 two months and giving up after losing 5 pounds?

Always Go the Healthy Route!

Diet and exercise will affect your body. Weight loss brings along chemical and physical changes as we go through the process. That's a good thing because our body is getting used to being lighter. It learns to run more efficiently and it is purging all the crap and garbage you used to put into it.

Exercise is great even if we don't need it to lose weight. I strongly urge everyone to adopt some form of exercise even if you are skinny. Exercise helps ward off some diseases and increase our ability to fight disease as well. Even if you can control your diet and lose weight without exercise, get some anyway. It is just smart and healthy to do that. You will feel better, sleep better and have more energy!

But along with the healthy route, use common sense and take your time as well. Do not stress your body and systems with a massive exercise program or very restricted diet on day one. Gradually ease your way into it and increase things over time.

Do this YOUR Way!

We have devised the CDO program in such a way that it can be YOUR program. You can decide how you want to proceed and what you want to do to achieve your results. This is all about what is right for you NOT anyone else.

Some people love to exercise. They can run marathons and compete in triathlons and other stuff. That might not be who you are or what you are capable of. Don't let anyone control what you do or how you lose weight but YOU!

People try to be helpful but everyone is different. Find the perfect balance between diet and exercise and behaviors that works for you. Once you find it, stick with it. Change it as you need to but stick with it. Long Term weight loss does not occur with 4 months of dieting and then a return to what made you heavy in the first place. It is by finding out what is right for you and then making that your life long behavior that results in losing weight and keeping it off.

Be Flexible!

Weigh loss is a constantly varying process. It's kind of nature's way of never letting you get too comfortable.

As you lose weight and your body starts to work better, you burn less calories and have to work a little harder. It might sound cruel but it really is a good thing.

That means that what worked so well a month ago might not work that well today. So we need to monitor things and make little adjustments. Or we just need to realize and understand what it going on and not get discouraged.

Maybe you were losing 3 pounds a week and that has no slowed to 1 pound a week. We either make an adjustment or we let ourselves know that 1 pound a week is still going in the right direction and will still lead us to our goal. We should NOT expect to keep up a certain level of weight loss throughout the entire program. But we should expect to understand what is going on and either modify things or accept them.

Never be afraid to try new things or even a new approach. If you think of something new, and it seems to make sense, give it a try! Just monitor your results to see how things are going. Success is often achieved by people who are willing to change course in mid stream when conditions call for it. CDO is all about doing what works for you no matter what that might be!

Take Time to Enjoy the Process

Whether you are trying to lose 5 pounds or 100 pounds, what you are doing is a very good and positive thing.

You should congratulate yourself on making the effort each and every day. Celebrate the loss of every pound and track your progress towards your goal.

Do not look at this process as a negative thing. Our minds hate negative things and tend to avoid them. Instead, enjoy the process and tell yourself every day that you are closer to your goal than you were last week this time. Anything that you can do to keep a positive approach and attitude will help you achieve your goal.

Keeping a positive outlook also helps you keep up the effort for a longer period of time. Eventually everything you are doing will become habit and require little or no thought. But until that happens, we need to stay motivated and focused on our end goal. Staying positive greatly helps us do just that.

Keep Focused

Speaking of keeping focused, we always should know where we are, where we are going and where we have been. There will be times when we have a bad day or a bad week and maybe our hearts just aren't in it for some reason. It happens to everyone from time to time.

But if we can say to ourselves "Hey, I lost 1 pound this week and I am only 15 pounds from my goal. I have lost 19 pounds since I started this two months ago!" all of this helps keep us excited, motivated and focused.

That is why we concentrated and pushed knowledge so much in these pages. The more we know the easier it is to stay focused. The more we understand, the easier it is to keep focused on our objectives and the more focused we are on things the easier and faster it is to adapt to changes and bumps in the road.

Accept Setbacks

Setbacks will happen. We talk about them in another chapter. But always keep focused on the good that you have accomplished and what brought you all that success. Sometimes over time we get distracted or start doing little things that undermine our efforts. Getting back to basics and what brought you success before is the best way to get back on track!

Laugh a Little!

The world would be a far better place if only people would learn to laugh a little bit more. Everyone is so serious and everyone is so focused on little things that they lose focus of the big picture.

Life without laughter or humor is a barren lifestyle. We need to make sure we take the time to enjoy ourselves and laugh a little bit. Weight loss is no different. If you want to go out and have some fun, then do it.

Don't take yourself so seriously either. Be able to laugh at your mistakes and take joy in your successes and learn from your failures. Not only will it help you become a better person, it will help you relax and stay focused as well.

The things you do to control life's stresses will go a long way in enabling you to navigate through life without the problems so many people have these days. I see people who have all the money in the world still consumed with making more while life passes them by. People who have everything going for them yet cannot relax and enjoy the life they have created.

When it comes to weight, strive to be the weight you feel comfortable at. Unless there is a medical reason, strive to be the person that looks and acts like you want to. Keep in mind that there is a health component attached to weight gain and loss and you must always be aware of that. But take time to live the life you want and be willing to laugh not only at others but at yourself as well.

Life is just too short to be dominated by BS!

Dealing with Setbacks

It's not a question of if you are going to have a setback. It's just a question of when it is going to happen. There are so many outside influences and situations that a setback is almost guaranteed to happen. So the question is not "Will I have a setback?" but rather "How do I deal with the setback when it occurs?"

There are a few things we need to understand about setbacks.

First, Setbacks are not Necessarily Failures.

If we abandon our diet and exercise plan intentionally and gain 5 pounds, then that would be considered a failure. But if we have a setback because of outside situations and events, then that would be a different situation.

People are creatures of habit and as long as we control what we do, when we do it, and how we do it then we are in our comfort zone. But when something happens where we lose control, setbacks often occur.

A prime example are the holidays. During the holidays our lives are different. There are holiday parties, holiday foods and an abundance of holiday snacks, getting together and, of course, those holiday meals. These can take us out of our comfort zone and get us into trouble. In the same group would be weddings, birthday parties and other similar events.

If we put on a few pounds, or just break even, over the holiday period, some people get upset or depressed. That is just foolish. The right way to look at it is to accept what had happened, chalk it up to holiday celebration, and move on.

Vacations are another time when you might cut yourself a little bit of slack and go outside your plan a LITTLE. Maybe your goal for a vacation is to end your vacation at the same weight as you started. If you are going on a cruise or some other food based vacation, then maybe allowing yourself to gain a couple of pounds over the week is not such a bad thing either. Again, I said a few pound. Not 10 or 20 pounds!

Second, Sometimes Conditions Prohibit Weight Loss

When you are not feeling well or when you are sick, it is not advisable to continue eating or exercising like you normally would.

In some cases, the body feels so bad that you simply cannot do those things.

This is not a failure. This is simply being smart and realizing that this is a time to heal your body not push it to lose weight. The key to these time frames is to eat well but responsibly. Increase your calorie intake to give your body the power to heal itself. But the body does not heal well through hot fudge sundaes! Eat more healthy foods like soups and vegetable to build strength and a good immune system.

In other words, allow yourself this downtime and ready yourself to start back up when you are feeling better. When you do start up again after a sickness gradually work your way into it. Consult your doctor after an illness and ask them when it is safe to continue.

Third, Sometimes Work Gets in the Way!

Some of us work in offices or have jobs where we must entertain clients or routinely take customers or others out for lunch or dinner. In these lunches and dinners it is often not reasonable to sit down with just a salad while everyone else is scarfing down a big steak.

But that does not mean you have an excuse to eat like a pig, either! Pick a healthy entrée like boiled chicken and a salad or something lower in calories. It is still possible to fit in and still eat somewhat healthy at the same time.

Work and social responsibilities are things that need to be factored into our weight loss plan.

If you know they are going to happen, you can plan for them and make changes to integrate them into your plan.

Maybe it means eating less on other days or increasing your exercise. Whatever the changes might be, if you know they are coming, you can prepare for them!

Fourth, Sometimes Failures ARE Failures

If you are reading this and you are human, raise your hand. OK, now that we know that everyone reading this book is human we can safely say that we all make mistakes and we all have lapses in judgment. That being said, this is not about blame, it is about working through a setback and getting back on track.

When we experience a setback it is important to understand what we did to cause it and how we might do something differently next time we are in that same situation. Sometimes there will be nothing we could have done or should have done and that is fine as well. But most of the time there will be something we could have done differently that would have lead to a different result.

If we are unable to adhere to our goals and plans because they are simply too much for us, then we need to adjust those plans and goals so that we can continue to follow those plans. But if it is just that we are unwilling to do what is necessary, then that is something else entirely.

Lack of motivation is one of the most common reasons for failing to lose weight.

If we say we want to lose weight but continue to wolf down burgers, fries, milkshakes and other similar type foods, no diet or exercise plan is going to work. We need to have some level of commitment in order to succeed.

If you are having trouble sticking to your plan, and if adjustments to your plan are not enough, then perhaps we need to spend some time getting back to why we started down this road in the first place. Get back to your roots and the reasons you wanted to lose weight in the first place.

Ask yourself if you are closer to your goal now than you were when you started. Ask yourself if you feel better now than you did before. In other words, search for positive things that you have noticed so far from your weight loss to see if those things can motivate you to start back up again. Very often you just need to re-find your source of motivation to get back on track.

When Nothing Seems to Work

Weight loss seems to be a very straightforward process. When you burn more calories than you take in, you lose weight. But despite something so simple, sometimes things get in the way and progress is slow or seemingly impossible.

When this occurs, we need to look for answers. This is not meant to assess blame but merely to highlight possible things that are the cause of our problem. That way we can either resign ourselves to the reality of the situation or move forward to make the needed changes.

Her are some common reasons why people fail to lose weight:

Medical Issues

Everything we talked about in the book assumes one very important thing.

We assumed that your body is working the way it normally should. But that might not be the case. It is entirely possible that your body is doing something that causes weight gain.

That could be a metabolic or glandular issue or any number of possible causes. That is why it is so critical to get your doctor involved with your weight loss. They can help you pinpoint medical issues or they might even be aware of certain things in your medical history that could cause your inability to lose weight.

It might be as simple as getting a prescription to help you lose weight. **NOTE: This is NOT the same thing as taking weight loss supplement and over the counter weight loss products!**

Emotional Issues

Sometimes we might not want to admit it but our brains can be standing in the way of our weight loss. The human mind is very complex and sometimes issues and emotional trauma create problems with us in everyday life and that includes weight loss.

"Emotional Eating" is one classic issue where people resort to food for comfort and stress release. This leads to overeating, binge eating and high consumption of high calorie and high fat comfort foods.

If you suspect that you suffe3r from such a condition, or any other emotional issue, we urge you to seek counseling. Even if you do manage to lose the weight, if you still have the emotional issues chances are you will gain it all back again in the future.

Getting help is not a sign of weakness or anything you should be ashamed of. Instead, you should be commended for taking action and for wanting to make your life better. Have a consultation with a behavioral therapist to see what issue you might have that need to be addressed. Your emotional health is every bit as important as your physical health. In a lot of ways the two are intertwined and emotional health will effect physical well being.

Lack of Honesty

This is a tough one to deal with at times. When it comes to losing weight, there is a LOT of honesty involved. If you are not honest with yourself, the information you used to create your plan will not be accurate and the result is a plan that will not work as well as it should.

If you tell yourself you are reducing your diet by 1,000 a day when in reality you are reducing it only 100 calories, something will suffer. The same goes for exercise. If you tell yourself you are getting 1,500 calories burned off every day through exercise and the real figure is 100, your weight loss will suffer.

We all want to get results with as little effort as possible. But honesty plays a huge role in identifying problems, making decisions and designing plans. If you cannot be honest with yourself, that will be a problem for you.

The great thing about being dishonest with yourself is that things can change immediately once you start being honest. At any point in time you can stop lying to yourself and be honest.

You can gather accurate and truthful data and create an accurate and success based plan to follow. You can go from failure to success literally overnight once you start being honest with yourself. Always remember that the only one who needs to know about the data you gather and your weight loss plan is YOU. No one else needs to know! (Except for your doctor who you always should be honest with anyway....)

Lack of Commitment

This is another area where many people suffer and have trouble. Mostly this occurs with people who are trying to lose weight because someone else told them to or wants them to. In other words, it's not something they have an interest in. It's something they are doing to make someone else happy.

This rarely works. Unless YOU want to lose the weight for a reason that is important to you, it will be hard to continue to do the things you are used to doing. You will resent the need for exercise and you will resent not eating everything you did before. Chances are the first chance you get you will stop.

As interesting as this might sound, even your doctor telling you that you have to lose weight for medical reasons will not be enough unless YOU believe them and want to change. This is similar to the person who smokes 3 packs a day whose doctor tells them they need to quit. If they don't want to quit, they ain't gonna!

The only way to overcome lack of commitment is to find a reason that is important to you to lose the weight. Maybe you feel a little better now that you lost a few pounds and can build on that. Maybe your clothes fit better or you look better. Whatever you can find that is positive to build on, use it! Find a reason to continue that strikes a chord within you so that you can build a level of commitment you need to be successful.

Lack of Support

Most people need some kind of help in order to achieve a long term goal. With weight loss, this is even more important since our environment is one of the most important factors.

If your family insists on having fatty food and rich desserts around all the time and eat them in your presence, it is going to make things that much harder for you. If the food is there staring you in the face, eventually you are going to be tempted to eat it. Once you start, it becomes a real slippery slope.

The same goes for your work environment. If people there are always snacking and bringing high calorie foods to you to snack on, eventually you will eat some. After all, a person can stand only so much temptation.

We need to surround ourselves with people who will support us. People who will respect our efforts enough to keep bad foods out of our sight and encourage us to keep going.

People who will accompany us on walks or play a set of tennis with us. In other words, people who will be a positive influence on us.

If we cannot find those people, we might have no choice other than to change our environment and try to stay from those people who try to get us to stop trying to lose weight. It can be a tough decision but most of the time we can make it work. Nicely tell people how much this means to you and ask them for their help or co-operation. Don't expect them to give up the foods they love, just ask them to keep them out of your view and environment.

Weight Loss Tips

Do eat low calorie foods like fruits and vegetables

Do eat regularly scheduled meals and snacks. Do not skip meals.

Do get regular aerobic exercise

Do make your doctor part of your weight loss plan

Do make sure you are healthy enough for diet and exercise

Do try to lose weight for YOU, not because someone else wants you to.

Do moderate your efforts and diet.

Do everything in a healthy and responsible fashion
 Do drink water to stay hydrated.

Do ask others for their support and
assistance

Do your best to stick with your weight loss plan

Do be honest with yourself while setting goals and making choices

Do take time to celebrate success and achieving your goals

Do take time to remind yourself of the benefits of losing weight

Do stay focused and motivated no matter what it takes.

Do adjust or change goals as conditions require

Do your best. No one can ask for anything more.

Do lose weight at a responsible and healthy rate.

Do monitor your progress frequently to catch problems early

Do address and resolve behavioral issues that lead you to eat.

Weight Loss Things to Avoid!

Don't Skip Meals

Don't cut back on water

Don't reduce your calories per day to starvation levels

Don't do more exercise than you can safely do

Don't try and lose weight too fast!

Don't try to do everything all at once

Don't skip steps in your plan

Don't resort to dangerous fad diets or diet products
Don't do anything that you feel is unhealthy

Don't ignore doctors advice or warnings

NEVER purge yourself after eating! NEVER!

Don't do anything to excess. Always use moderation

Don't get discouraged. Practice patience and discipline

Don't expect things to change without a behavior change.

Don't ignore aches and pains or hurt when exercising.

Don't exercise the same body parts every day. Let them heal.

Don't forget to stretch before exercising and cool down after.

Don't try and do it alone. Ask for help and support from others.

Don't be stubborn! Adjust goals and plans as things change

Don't Give Up!!!!!!!

Conclusion

We find ourselves now at a crossroads. We have provided you with information to help you be successful at losing your weight. We have guided you through creating a flexible plan suited to your need to get you started. But now the time for planning has stopped. At least for now.

Now it is up to you.

It is up to you to follow the plan you have created.

It is up to you to monitor your results and make changes as you need them.

It is up to you to create a supportive environment and ask family and friends for their support.

It is up to you to get some more exercise.

It is up to you to stay on a healthy diet and a healthy lifestyle.

It is up to you to follow things through to make it all work.

Sometimes it will be fun and you will see great results. Other times you might hit a rough patch and get a little discouraged. But never lose sight of your goals or lose your motivation.

Look inside of you for your motivation. Discover how much better you feel each and every day as the pounds come off and your conditioning improves. Take pride and enjoyment is being able to do something today that you might not have been able to do a few months ago.

This is all for you. This is all about making your life richer, better and more fulfilling. It is about being able to do more of what you want and living a longer and healthier life.

Your weight is more than a number on a scale. It is a reflection of your health and well being. Don't lose weight for anyone else. Lose it for you. Lose it so you are around longer and can experience more in your life.

When you look at weight loss in this way, it makes the work and sacrifice so much easier. Try it, you'll see.

Good luck on your weight loss efforts.

CDO Weight Loss Calculation Sheet

To Figure Calorie Reduction Needed to Stabilize Weight Gain:

Average Weight Gain per week in pounds:

_____

Multiply above answer by 3,500:

_____

This is the number of calories you will have to reduce in order to stabilize your weight at its current level.

To Figure Calorie Reduction Required to Lose Weight:

Enter the number of pounds you wish to lose every week (ideally 1-2 lbs): _____

Multiply the above answer by 3,500 calories:

_____

This is the number of calories that you will have to reduce or burn off in addition to the calories (if any) in the first section to lose the amount of weight you wish to lose each week.

To figure Total Number of Calories Required to Reach Your Goal:

Enter the amount of calorie reduction needed to stabilize current weight: _____

Enter the amount of calorie reduction needed to lose weight: _____

Add the two calorie totals here: _____

This is the number of calories you will have to reduce or burn to achieve your overall weekly weight loss goal.

To Figure the Amount of Calorie Reduction Through Diet Needed:

Enter total number of calories needed here: _____

Enter the number of calories burned through additional* exercise here: _____

Subtract the bottom number from the top number: _____

This is the number of calories you need to reduce your current diet by to lose weight and achieve your goals.

To Figure Amount of Exercise Needed:

Enter total Calories Here:

_____

Enter calorie reduction through diet Here:

_____

Subtract to get calories needed to burn:

_____

*Additional exercise means the amount of NEW exercise you need to do in order to increase the number of calories burned. Do NOT count exercise you already have been doing. For example, if you run 5 miles a week now and you increase that to 10 miles a week, then you would only count 5 miles for your new exercise! Enter only the NEW things you will be doing to lose weight.

www.ingramcontent.com/pod-product-compliance
Lightning Source LLC
Chambersburg PA
CBHW071154290526
45787CB00001BA/384